Contents

Preface

The Pediatric Adolescent Gynecology (PAG) program at the University of Louisville was founded by Dr. Joseph S. Sanfilippo and has been one of the premier training programs in this specialty since its inception in 1990. It has trained fellows including Drs Hertweck and Perlman, as well as residents, medical and nurse practitioner students in all of the primary care (Pediatrics, Med-Peds, and Family Medicine) specialties as well as those of Gynecology and Reproductive Endocrinology.

This book provides a comprehensive review of all of the common and less encountered PAG problems that patients present to us on a daily basis, both in the ambulatory as well as the surgical setting. This is not just a review but also more a basic handbook on how to assess these problems quickly and efficiently, enabling the clinician to determine and execute a management plan. The book is designed to be an easy to follow how-to-guide for the most simple to the most complex problem. We completed a review of the literature, combined it with our clinical experience and placed the information in a bulleted text format with helpful photographs, figures and algorithms to assist both the student and the practitioner more easily care for the PAG patient.

Hence, in this text, the reader will find diagnostic and treatment methodology for the most simple PAG problems such as vulvovaginitis and labial adhesions; for common issues like menstrual disorders and contraception; and for rare and more complex disorders such as Turner syndrome and ambiguous genitalia – with everything in-between.

We are grateful to Parthenon Publishing for recognizing the need for such a textbook. We are appreciative of the technical support as well as medical editing Leta Weedman has provided. We thank Drs. Pam Clark, Jacqueline Sugarman, Charles Maxfield, Dennis O'Connor (Pediatric Surgical Associates) and Claire Templeman for their expert review. We are indebted to our colleagues, especially our fellows and partners in the Department of Obstetrics and Gynecology and Women's Health for covering some of our clinical duties so that we could complete this book in a timely fashion. And finally to our assistants, especially Laura Lukat-Coffman, thank you for your constant support and for making it possible for us to get through our days in the allotted time.

Dedication

We dedicate this book to our families who allowed us the privilege of putting our experience on paper and gave us the encouragement to be the physicians that we are today.

1 Ambiguous genitalia (intersex disorder)

DEFINITION

Anatomic variation of the external genitalia making sex determination difficult

Characterized by clitoromegaly and labial fusion

Most cases present in the newborn, not in the adolescent

EVALUATION

This is a medical and social emergency in the newborn

75% of these cases have life-threatening salt wasting nephropathy that if unrecognized can cause hypotension, vascular collapse, and death

(1) First priority: ensure electrolyte/endocrinologic abnormalities corrected

- Check serum electrolytes

(2) Second priority: establish the most probable cause

- Inform parents of spectrum existing between virilized and feminized genitalia

(3) Postpone making a gender assignment

- Reassure parents: 'You have a healthy baby, but the external genitalia are incompletely developed and tests are necessary to determine the sex'
- Refer to the infant as 'the baby' rather than a boy or girl
- Instruct parents on how to deal with grandparents, sibs, babysitters and others who might note the child's genital appearance (e.g. 'The baby is different but normal and when the child is older he or she and the doctors will do what seems best')

DIFFERENTIAL DIAGNOSIS

(Based on histology of the gonad)

(1) Female pseudohermaphroditism: two ovaries – 46,XX karyotype

- Most common cause of ambiguous genitalia: congenital adrenal hyperplasia (CAH)
- Highest frequency in people of European Jewish, Hispanic, Italian, or Slavic descent
- Results from enzymatic defect in conversion of cholesterol to cortisol

    21-hydroxylase enzyme deficiency occurs in 95% cases

    These patients have:

    > elevated 17-hydroxyprogesterone (17-OHP)

    > low cortisol

    > elevated adrenocorticotropic hormone (ACTH)

    Other adrenal enzyme deficiencies rarely present at birth

    If female pseudohermaphrodite with unclear etiology:

    > Perform ACTH stimulation test with other precursor levels:

    >> 11-deoxycorticosterone

    >> 11-deoxycortisol

    >> 17-hydroxypregnenolone

(2) Male pseudohermaphroditism: two testes – 46,XY karyotype

- Types:

    > 80% have androgen receptor disorder with normal testosterone levels

    > 20% have inadequate testosterone production or are deficient in 5 alpha-reductase activity (the enzyme converting testosterone (T) to active form, dihydrotestosterone (DHT))

(3) True hermaphroditism: ovary and/or testis and/or ovotestis

- Very rare
- Chromosomal pattern frequency 46,XX > 46,XY mosaic > 46,XY
- Has both ovarian and testicular tissue

    Three categories:

    lateral – testis on one side, ovary on other

unilateral – ovotestis on one side, normal gonad on other

bilateral – two ovotestes

(4) Mixed gonadal dysgenesis:

- Second most common of ambiguous genitalia in newborn
- 45,X/46,XY mosaic pattern
- Characteristics:

  Testis on one side/streak gonad on other *or*

  Unilateral unicornuate uterus/fallopian tube on streak gonad side *or*

  Contralateral testis is dysgenetic/non-sperm producing

DIAGNOSTIC WORKUP

History

In the adolescent, when was ambiguity first noted?

Any pubertal signs? Breast or pubic hair development?

Family history:

- A family history of genital ambiguity, infertility, or unexpected changes at puberty may suggest a genetically transmitted trait

  Remember: Recessive traits tend to occur in siblings, while X-linked abnormalities tend to appear in males who are scattered sporadically across the family history
- Any possible consanguinity increases the likelihood of autosomal recessive disorders (e.g. CAH)
- A family history of neonatal deaths may suggest a previously missed diagnosis of CAH
- Although extremely rare, a history of maternal virilization may suggest an androgen-producing tumor

Pregnancy history:

- Any prior pregnancies with ambiguity
- Any prior pregnancies that ended in fetal demise/early death
- Any possible consanguinity
- Any hormonal ingestion/pharmaceutical exposure during pregnancy particularly androgens or progestational drugs
- Any maternal history of virilization or CAH

Physical examination

Overall assessment:

- Look for abnormal facial appearance or other dysmorphic features suggesting a multiple malformation syndrome (e.g. IUGR, abnormal body proportions)
- Look for abnormal skin pigmentation from high ACTH
- Look for evidence of salt wasting: decreased skin turgor, tears when crying
- In adolescents look for evidence of hirsutism

Breast development:

- Check Tanner staging (see Gynecologic examination, Chapter 21)

Abdomen:

- In adolescents: evaluate for male escutcheon
- Evaluate for masses

Gonadal examination:

- Palpate labioscrotal tissue for presence of gonadal tissue

  In infants, may need an assistant to hold infant still with thighs abducted. Start with fingers at line of inguinal canal and sweep down the canal on each side above the inguinal line. Any gonad that is nudged down toward the scrotum should be gently grasped by the other examining hand, noting the size and consistency of the gonadal tissue

- Note number of gonads, size, symmetry and position

  Palpable gonads below the inguinal canal are almost always a testicle and exclude diagnoses of gonadal female (e.g. CAH), Turner syndrome and pure gonadal dysgenesis

  Impalpable gonads even in an apparently virilized female infant should raise the possibility of a severely virilized female pseudohermaphrodite with CAH

External genitalia:

- Phallus: note the size and degree of differentiation, variations may represent clitoromegaly or hypospadias
- Urethral meatus: note position (on the glans, shaft or at perineum)
- Labioscrotal folds: are they separated or are they fused at the midline, giving an appearance of a scrotum. Rugose scrotal or labioscrotal folds with increased pigmentation suggest the possibility of increased corticotropin levels as part of the adrenogenital syndrome of CAH
- Vaginal introitus: is there an obvious normal opening

Rectal assessment:

- Evaluate for palpable cervix and uterus confirming internal mullerian structures. The uterus is relatively enlarged in the newborn secondary to maternal estrogenization, thereby permitting easy identification

Laboratory evaluation

Assess and follow serum electrolytes

- Look for high K, low Na

Measure serum 17-OHP level (may need serial measurements since higher levels occur during the first two days of life)

- Normal range = 82 to 400 ng/dl (3- to 5-day-olds). If > 400 ng/dl indicates CAH
- If 200–300 ng/dl, do ACTH stimulation test

Measure urinary 17-ketosteroids

- Normal range ≤ 1 mg/24 h

Measure serum cortisol, ACTH, dehydroepiandrosterone (DHEA), testosterone, DHT and T:DHT ratio

Chromosomal analysis (karyotype or fluorescence *in situ* hybridization for sex chromosome material)

Radiographic imaging (see Radiologic imaging for gynecologic conditions, Chapter 52)

- Abdominal and pelvic ultrasound
- Genitogram: retrograde injection of contrast material via the urogenital orifice
- Consider MRI in cases in which ultrasound or genitogram not definitive

May need endoscopic evaluation of urethra or urogenital sinus

Rarely need laparotomy or laparoscopy for gonadal biopsy

See Figure 1-1

Laboratory findings

If elevated 17-OHP with 46,XX karyotype: diagnosis is 21-hydroxylase deficiency

If normal 17-OHP with 46,XX karyotype and an unclear etiology, perform an ACTH stimulation test checking other steroid precursor levels (11-deoxycorticosterone, 11-deoxycortisol, 17-hydroxypregnenolone) to determine if another adrenal enzymatic defect is present

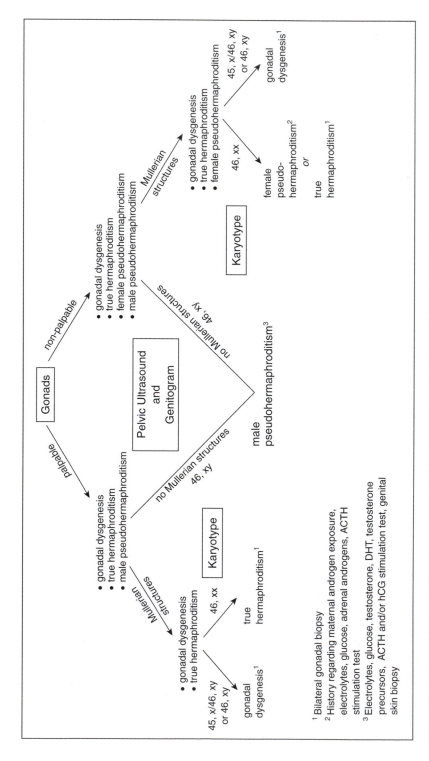

Figure 1-1 An approach to the evaluation of ambiguous genitalia in the newborn. ACTH, adrenocorticotropic hormone; DHT, dihydrotestosterone; hCG, human chorionic gonadotropin. With permission from Meyers-Seifer CH, Charest NJ. Diagnosis and management of patients with ambiguous genitalia. *Semin Perinatol* 1992:16:332–9. © 1992 Elsevier, Inc.

If patient is 46,XY with no mullerian structures and low testosterone or elevated T:DHT ratio: diagnosis is 5-alpha reductase deficiency

If normal 17-OHP and normal ACTH: diagnosis is either true hermaphroditism or gonadal dysgenesis

TREATMENT

Patients with ambiguous genitalia are best managed in a medical center with a full multidisciplinary team including:

Geneticist/genetic counselor

Endocrinologist

Surgeon

Obstetrician/gynecologist

Pediatric urologist

Psychologist

Treatment is based on underlying cause:

(1) Female pseudohermaphroditism

In CAH:

Goal is to replace deficient steroids while minimizing adrenal sex hormone and glucocorticoid excess, prevent virilization, optimize growth, protect potential fertility

Lifelong steroid and mineralocorticoid replacement with CAH required

- In infancy/childhood: hydrocortisone (HCT) 10–15 mg/m^2/day divided 3x/daily

    Use divided or crushed tablets of HCT

    Oral solution not recommended

- Monitor baby's weight, electrolytes, fluid status, plasma renin activity (salt-losing not manifested until day 6 to 14 of life)

    Decreased serum sodium, decreased aldosterone, elevated plasma renin indicate salt-losing condition. Need to add salt (2–4 g/day) to formula and add fludrocortisone acetate (Florinef, Apothecon, Princeton, NJ) 0.05–0.1 mg/day

- Stress dosing is 2–3 times the maintenance glucocorticoid dose

- Give stress dose with fever > 38.3°C (> 101°F), when vomiting or unable to take p.o. feeds, with trauma and before surgery

(2) Male pseudohermaphroditism/pure pseudohermaphroditism/mixed gonadal dysgenesis

If testicular tissue is intraabdominal: requires excision due to increased risk of malignancy with intraabdominal testes

(3) True hermaphroditism

Consult multi-disciplinary team for management

Surgical care

Postpone immediate surgical correction of the external genitalia in the newborn unless physically/medically necessary

Intraabdominal testicular tissue is at increased risk of malignancy and requires excision

Note: Appearances of genitalia during childhood are of less importance than functionality and post-pubertal erotic sensitivity of the genitalia; thus, surgery can potentially impair sexual or erotic function. Sexual development of the brain is influenced by androgens, which play a significant role in the etiology of gender identity; therefore, even CAH patients may develop a male gender identity. As such, clitoral surgery/sex reassignment might best be delayed until puberty or until a patient can make informed consent. Genital reconstruction may be unwise until the patient has had multiple longitudinal gender identity assessments (perhaps until as old as 8 or 9 years of age). Gender identity will most likely be discernible by that age, and puberty is unlikely to have commenced, thus all organs will still be intact. This decision is best made with consultation of a multi-disciplinary team of clinicians experienced with this condition.

BIBLIOGRAPHY

Consensus statement on 21-hydroxylase deficiency from The Lawson Wilkins Pediatric Endocrine Society and The European Society for Paediatric Endocrinology. *J Clin Endocrinol Metab* 2002;87:4048–53

Diamond M, Sigmuncson HK. Management of intersexuality: Guidelines for dealing with persons with ambiguous genitalia. *Arch Pediatr Adolesc Med* 1997;151:1046–50

Donohoe PK, Schnitzer JJ. Evaluation of the infant who has ambiguous genitalia, and principles of operative management. *Semin Pediatr Surg* 1996;5:30-40

Holm IA. Ambiguous genitalia in the newborn. In Emans SJ, Laufer MR, Goldstein DP, eds. *Pediatric and Adolescent Gynecology*. 4th edn. Philadelphia: Lippincott-Raven, 1998

Hutcheson J. Ambiguous genitalia and intersexuality. August 6, 1992:
http://www.emedicine.com/PED/topic1492.htm

Meyers-Seifer CH, Charest NJ. Diagnosis and management of patients with ambiguous genitalia. *Semin Perinatol* 1992;16:332–9

Reiner WG. Assignment of sex in neonates with ambiguous genitalia. *Curr Opin Pediatr* 1999;11:363

Slaughenhoupt BL. Diagnostic evaluation and management of the child with ambiguous genitalia. *J Ky Med Assoc* 1997;95:135–41

2 Amenorrhea

PRIMARY AMENORRHEA

DEFINITION

No menses by age 14 in absence of secondary sexual characteristics, *or*

No menses by 2 years after completing sexual development, *or*

No menses by age 16 regardless of secondary sexual characteristics

KEY POINTS

Menstruation is dependent on:

- An intact central nervous system (CNS) with appropriate hypothalamic–pituitary output
- Proper end-organ or ovarian responsiveness
- An intact outflow tract (normal functioning endometrium and patent uterus, cervix, and vagina)

Therefore, look for defect in one of the above in the history and physical exam (e.g. check for breast development and presence or absence of the uterus)

DIAGNOSIS

History

Assess intact central nervous system (CNS) or for any CNS symptoms

- Ask about anosmia, headaches, nausea, visual changes
- History of head trauma, CNS irradiation

Assess development of secondary sexual characteristics (end-organ response)

- At what age did breast development/pubic hair begin?
- Breast buds present on average by age 9.5 years in African Americans; by age 10.4 in Caucasians
- Pubic hair present on average by age 9.4 in African Americans; by age 10.6 in Caucasians

Assess for outflow obstructive symptoms

- Does the patient have cyclic abdominal pain?

Physical examination

Check height and weight and plot on growth curves

Evaluate growth curves to see any growth trend (e.g. persistent height < 5th percentile might indicate Turner syndrome or a growth disorder)

Check for presence of breast tissue and uterus to plan further management strategy

Check perineum to ensure patent outflow tract (is hymen patent?) and determine presence of uterus

Evaluate for transverse vaginal septa by placing single digit into vagina to palpate cervix or place small Huffman specula into vaginal opening to visualize cervix (rule out cervical agenesis)

MANAGEMENT

If imperforate hymen: see Hymenal anatomy (Chapter 25)

If transverse vaginal septa: see Vaginal tract abnormalities (Chapter 66)

If breasts absent/uterus present (see Figure 2-1):

- Indicates lack of estrogen
- Either from hypothalamic–pituitary-ovarian (HPO) failure or gonadal failure (see Premature ovarian failure, Chapter 47)

If breasts present/uterus absent (see Figure 2-2):

- Breast development indicates estrogen production
- Uterine absence indicates congenital absence or androgen insensitivity

If breasts absent/uterus absent (see Figure 2-3):

- Lack of breasts indicates lack of estrogen production
- Either from gonadal dysgenesis/agonadism/or rare gonadal deficiencies
- Lack of uterus indicates gonadal production of Mullerian inhibiting substance

If breasts present/uterus present/normal patent hymen: evaluate and manage as per secondary amenorrhea

- Presence of breasts indicates estrogen production at some point

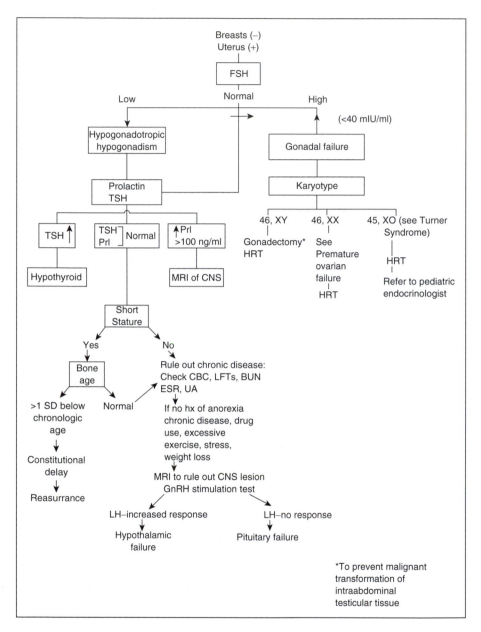

Figure 2-1   Management algorithm for primary amenorrhea when breasts are absent and uterus is present. BUN, blood urea nitrogen; CBC, complete blood count; CNS, central nervous system; ESR, erythrocyte sedimentation rate; FSH, follicle stimulating hormone; GnRH, gonadotropin releasing hormone; HRT, hormone replacement therapy; LFTs, liver function tests; LH, luteinizing hormone; MRI, magnetic resonance imaging; Prl, prolactin; TSH, thyroid stimulating hormone; UA, urinalysis

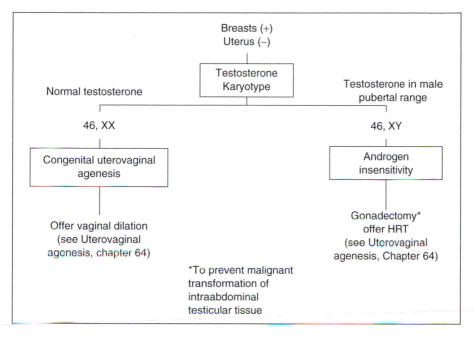

Figure 2-2   Management algorithm for primary amenorrhea when breasts are present and uterus is absent. HRT, hormone replacement therapy

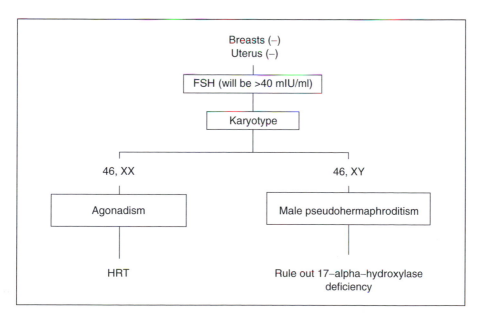

Figure 2-3   Management algorithm for primary amenorrhea when breasts are absent and uterus is absent. FSH, follicle stimulating hormone; HRT, hormone replacement therapy

SECONDARY AMENORRHEA

DEFINITION

Absence of menses for 3–6 months in previously menstruating women

KEY POINTS

Evaluate for specific causes of amenorrhea in girls with cycles > 90 days: (e.g. pregnancy, eating disorders, hypothalamic amenorrhea)

Most common cause of secondary amenorrhea is pregnancy

Persistent oligomenorrhea (cycles > 35 day intervals) requires evaluation

DIAGNOSIS

History

Menstrual history:

>   When did menarche occur (average age 12.4–12.8 years)?

>   When was last normal flow?

>   What was normal duration and flow of menses?

>   Any history of dysmenorrhea?

Review of past history:

>   Any chronic diseases? (e.g. Crohn's disease)

>   Any childhood illnesses?

>   Any childhood radiation treatment or chemotherapy?

>   Any past or current medication use?

>   Any past surgery?

>   Any surgery on the uterus (D & C)?

Review of symptoms:

>   Vasomotor symptoms (e.g. hot flashes indicative of a hypoestrogenic state)

>   Androgen excess signs (acne, hirsutism, etc.)

>   Galactorrhea (indicating prolactin excess)

>   Cyclic bloating/pain (indicating uterovaginal obstruction)

>   Headaches/fatigue/palpitations/nervousness (indicate thyroid dysfunction)

>   Visual changes/nausea (may be associated with CNS lesion)

Review of habits:

> Nutrition/what patient eats every day
>
> Recent weight loss/gain
>
> Amount of physical activity
>
> Recent changes in life/stressors (death, divorce, move)

Confidential sexual history:

> Does patient participate in any sexual activity (petting, oral–anal intercourse, vaginal–penile intercourse)?

Physical examination

Check patient's height/weight and plot on curves

- Look for significant weight increases/decreases or persistent < 5th percentile scores

Check pulse/blood pressure

- Look for bradycardia, hypotension that may be associated with anorexia
- Hypertension may be associated with androgen excess due to Cushing disease

Evaluate for signs of hirsutism

- Acne, facial hair, acanthosis nigricans of the neck, axilla

Fundoscopy, visual field and cranial nerve assessment

- Look for defects that may be associated with CNS tumor or lesion

Palpate thyroid

- Any enlargement of gland or asymmetry

Breast exam

- Sexual maturity rate development (Tanner stage)
- Palpate and evaluate for galactorrhea

Abdominal exam

- Check for masses, pregnancy, tenderness, striae
- Check for male escutcheon pubic hair pattern

Pelvic

- Sexual maturity rate pubic hair development (Tanner stage)
  - Excess hair may indicate androgen excess
  - Absent or sparse hair may indicate androgen insensitivity

- Check for clitoromegaly
- Evaluate for estrogen status of vagina

  Is the tissue estrogenized: pale pink with white normal discharge
- Are the uterus and ovaries normal size?
- Look for fissures, skin tags or perineal fistulas

  May indicate inflammatory bowel disease

MANAGEMENT

(see Figure 2-4)

Principles of management

Attempt to restore ovulatory function

If ovulation cannot be restored, estrogen–progesterone therapy is usually indicated

- Combined estrogen–progestin oral contraceptive pill *or*
- Conjugated estrogen 0.625 mg for days 1–25 with medroxyprogesterone acetate 10 mg daily for days 16–25

Many causes of amenorrhea require frequent re-evaluation

Specific causes of amenorrhea:

- Systemic disease/endocrinopathies

  Treat underlying disease and menses will return:

  Thyroid replacement with hypothyroidism

  Normalization of serum glucose in diabetes

  Surgical or medical treatment of prolactinoma/hyperprolactinemia

  Replace hormone deficit in cases of pituitary destruction/inadequacy

  Glucocorticoid replacement in congenital adrenal hyperplasia

  Addressing chronic disease issues

  Inflammatory bowel disease

  Correcting eating disorders with increased weight

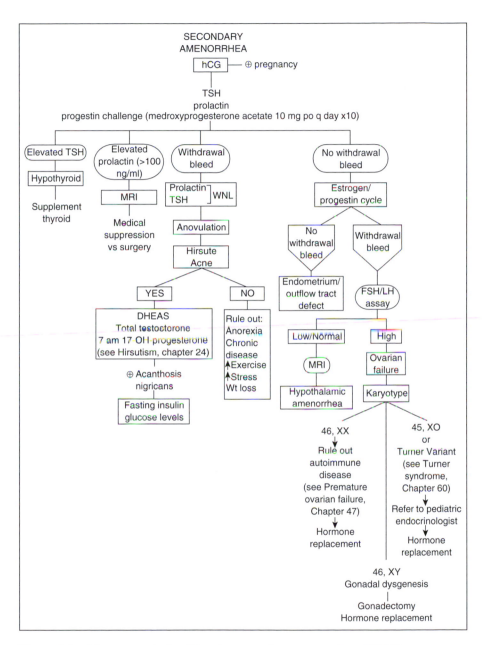

Figure 2-4 Management algorithm for secondary amenorrhea. DHEAS, dehydroepiandrosterone sulfate; FSH, follicle stimulating hormone; hCG, human chorionic gonadotropin; LH, luteinising hormone; MRI, magnetic resonance imaging; TSH, thyroid stimulating hormone; WNL, within normal limits

- Patients with ovarian failure:

  Will require hormone replacement as above

- Patients with polycystic ovarian syndrome:

  May require cyclic medroxyprogesterone acetate 10 mg po 12–14 days of month or oral contraceptive pills (see Polycystic ovarian syndrome, Chapter 45)

BIBLIOGRAPHY

Chumlea WC, Schubert CM, Roche AF, *et al*. Age at menarche and racial comparisons in US girls. *Pediatrics* 2003;111:110–13

Flug D. Menstrual patterns in adolescent Swiss girls: a longitudinal study. *Ann Hum Biol* 1984;11:495–508

Pletcher JR, Slap GB. Menstrual disorders: amenorrhea. *Pediatr Clin North Am* 1999;46:505–18

Treloar AE, Boynton RE, Behn BG, Brown BW. Variations in the human menstrual cycle through reproductive life. *Int J Fertil* 1967;12:77–126

Vollman RF. The menstrual cycle. In Friedman EA, ed. *Major Problems in Obstetrics and Gynecology*, vol 7. Philadelphia, PA: WB Saunders, 1977;1–191

WHO Task Force on Adolescent Reproductive Health. *J Adolesc Health Care* 1986;7:236–44

3 Bartholin's abscess

Results from occlusion of the main duct of the Bartholin's gland or small ductule

Abscess recognized with signs and symptoms of tenderness, swelling and erythema

INCISION AND DRAINAGE

Perform in a place where some type of sedation is available

Administer 1% xylocaine over the incision site at the most medial portion

Use 15-blade scalpel incision, not to exceed 2 mm (size of word Bartholin catheter)

Culture the drainage for *Neisseria gonorrhoeae, Chlamydia trachomatis* and aerobic/anaerobic bacteria

Break adhesions with sterile Q-tip or small forceps taking care not to extend incision

Irrigate the cavity with saline using a 16- or 18-gauge angiocath without the needle attached, to a 10–20 ml syringe

Insert the word catheter

Expand the balloon as directed per catheter instructions

FOLLOW-UP CARE

Sitz baths 3–4 times per week

Analgesia: Non-steroidal antiinflammatory drugs (NSAIDs), acetaminophen with codeine or with oxycodone

Return in one week. Drain some of the fluid out of the word catheter as needed. Remove at the end of two weeks

Treat the results of the cultures as indicated

If sexually transmitted disease (STD) culture(s) is positive, screen for all STDs including hepatitis, syphilis, and HIV (for treatment see Sexually transmitted diseases, Chapter 56)

Advise to place nothing in the vagina until healed

If this becomes recurrent without underlying cause then marsupialization is indicated

4 Breast abscess

May result from obstruction of mammary duct, irritation/abrasion of nipple and cellulitis of surrounding chest wall

Although may occur in the postpartum state, non-postpartum abscesses are more common

CAUSES

Neonatal abscess:

- Usually *Staphylococcus aureus*, but may have anaerobic bacteria in combination or as the primary etiology
- Beta-lactamase producing bacteria may be present in up to 50% of cases

Non-postpartum breast abscesses:

- Mixed flora

    S. aureus, *Bacteroides* spp. streptococcus Group B, *Escherichia coli*

Postpartum abscesses:

- *S. aureus*

DIAGNOSIS

History

Localized edema, erythema and pain of the breast

History of previous breast abscess

Associated symptoms of fever, vomiting, drainage from mass or nipple

Physical examination

Tender, indurated or fluctuant erythematous breast mass

Commonly in the areolar/periareolar area

+/– Fever and or axillary adenopathy

+/– Discharge from mass/nipple

Imaging

Breast ultrasound: to distinguish between cellulitis and blocked duct or abscess

MANAGEMENT

Children

Due to concern about damage to the breast bud complex, avoid needle aspiration of abscess – Use antibiotics first:

- Amoxicillin–clavulanate 20–40 mg/kg/day orally (every 12 hours in neonate/every 8 hours in children > 40 kg) for 2 weeks

If febrile, hospitalize with IV antibiotics and apply warm packs to breast bid every 48 hours

- Ampicillin–sulbactam sodium

    3 months to 12 years: 100–200 mg of ampicillin/kg/day IV (150–300 mg ampicillin–sulbactam sodium) divided q 6 hours

    If > 12 years: use adult dose

- Alternative antibiotics that cover beta-lactam producing *S. aureus/Bacteroides*: clindamycin, cefoxitin, imipenem

When afebrile 24 hours, continue treatment with oral antibiotics to complete 2 weeks of therapy

Reevaluate in 2 weeks after completion antibiotic therapy, and consider repeat ultrasound/exam 6–12 weeks post treatment to ensure complete resolution

Adolescents

Ultrasound guided aspiration:

- Apply topical anesthetic (see EMLA use, Chapter 17) or use subcutaneous lidocaine
- Aspirate abscess contents with 18-gauge needle attached to 10 ml syringe
- Send aspirate for cytology, aerobic and anaerobic culture and sensitivity

- Prescribe post-aspiration antibiotics for 14 days (need *Staphylococcus* and anaerobic coverage)

  Amoxicillin–clavulanate 500 mg po every 8 hours × 14 days

  or

  Clindamycin 300 mg po every 6 hours × 14 days

- Local care would include warm compresses bid vs hot shower to breast bid × 48 hours

- Prescribe post-aspiration pain medication: NSAIDs, Tylenol with codeine or Tylenol with oxycodone

If patient with systemic symptoms, consider IV antibiotics:

- 1.5 g (1 g ampicillin + 0.5 g sulbactam) to 3 g (2 g ampicillin + 1 g sulbactam) IV every 6 to 8 hours, not to exceed 4 g/day sulbactam or 8 g/day ampicillin

Follow-up twice weekly:

- Watch for recurrence, may need repeat aspiration or surgical incision and drainage especially when abscess > 3 cm diameter and/or volume of aspirated pus about 9 ml

- If abscess does not resolve, check culture and sensitivity results to ensure no antibiotic resistance and reevaluate patient as the cause may be an infected ectatic duct that may require excision of the obstructed lactiferous duct (microdochectomy)

Complications

Recurrent or persistent infection (40–50%)

- May require incision and drainage (I & D) under general anesthesia

Scarring

BIBLIOGRAPHY

Blumstein H. Breast abscesses and masses. July 5, 2001. http://www.emedicine.com/emrg/topic68.htm

Brooks I. The aerobic and anaerobic microbiology of neonatal breast abscess. *Pediatr Inf Dis J* 1991:10:785–6

Hook GW, Ikeda DM. Treatment of breast abscesses with US-guided percutaneous needle drainage without indwelling catheter placement. *Radiology* 1999;213: 579–82

Schwarz RJ, Shrestha R. Needle aspiration of breast abscesses. *Am J Surg* 2001;182: 117–19

5 Breast anomalies

CONGENITAL BREAST ANOMALIES

Accessory nipples (polythelia):

Prevalence: 2% of population

Diagnosis:

- Additional nipples anywhere along the milk line (see Figure 5-1)

Treatment:

- If in area of frequent trauma, can be excised surgically

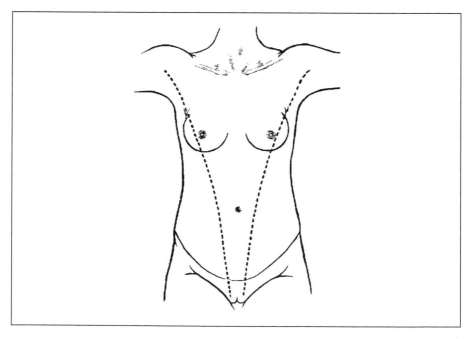

Figure 5-1 The 'milk line' corresponding to the embryologic mammary ridge. Accessory nipples, the most common congenital anomaly, and accessory breast tissue occur along these lines. With permission from Wiebke EA, Niederhuber JE. Disorders of the breast. In Carpenter SEK, Rock JA, eds. *Pediatric and Adolescent Gynecology*. Philadelphia, PA: Lippincott-Raven Publishers, 1996:418

Accessory breast tissue (polymastia):

May accompany polythelia

May have engorgement with lactation

Treatment:

- Rare need for surgical intervention – usually for cosmesis

Absence of nipple (athelia):

Treatment:

- Consult with plastic surgeon

Absence of breast tissue:

Uncommon – unilateral predominance

May occur with associated chest wall deformities:

- Poland's syndrome of aplasia of pectoralis muscles, rib deformities, webbed fingers, radial nerve aplasia
- Traumatic loss of breast bud (e.g. prior chest tube placement at bud site)

Treatment:

- Refer to plastic surgeon to correct

DEVELOPMENTAL BREAST ANOMALIES

Tuberous breasts:

Definition:

- Breast tissue limited in vertical and horizontal diameters at the base in association with an overdeveloped nipple–areolar complex (resembles a tuberous root plant)

Management:

- Plastic surgery consultation and correction
- May require tissue expansion in cases with skin deficiency
- Preferable to perform only single surgery therefore preferable to delay correction until breast development complete

Virginal/juvenile breast hypertrophy:

Definition:

- Pathologic overgrowth of breast tissue out of proportion to the body and chest size

Diagnosis:

- Usually occurs near menarche
- May be familial
- Evaluation should rule out presence of an underlying mass (e.g. giant fibroadenoma)

Treatment:

- Reduction mammoplasty in consultation with plastic surgery

BIBLIOGRAPHY

Templeman C, Hertweck SP. Breast disorders in the pediatric and adolescent patient. *Obstet Gynecol Clin North Am* 2000;27:19–34

6 Breast asymmetry

Neonatal:

> Unilateral or bilateral breast enlargement
>
> Secondary to maternal estrogen stimulation
>
> May have associated clear or cloudy nipple discharge
>
> Spontaneous resolution within 1st months of life
>
> Persistence requires evaluation for precocious puberty
>
> - Consider ultrasound to rule out cyst before referral to pediatric endocrinology

Adolescent:

> Common complaint at thelarche as the onset of breast development (thelarche) is often asymmetric
>
> Usually resolves by late adolescence
>
> 25% persist after age 18

History

> When did breast development (thelarche) begin?
>
> Compare thelarche temporally with onset of other sexual characteristics (e.g. pubic hair)
>
> Assess for symptoms of tenderness, erythema, discharge
>
> History of prior chest surgery/trauma/intravenous lines/chest tube placement
>
> (concern for interference with breast bud complex)
>
> History of congenital anomalies, scoliosis, familial breast disease

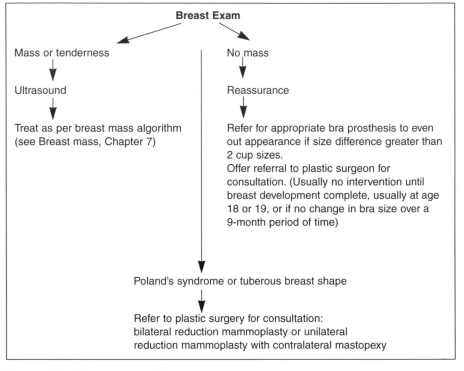

Figure 6-1   Management of breast asymmetry

Physical examination

Perform breast exam in sitting and reclining position

Check for absence of pectoralis major muscle on hypoplastic breast side, also called Poland's syndrome

- hypoplasia of pectoralis muscles, breast and areola
- anomalies of the rib cage, vertebral column, shoulder blade, armpit
- symbrachydactyly (short fingers with webbing in proximal portion)
- anomalies of the neurovascular structures of ipsilateral arm
- hypoplasia of the hand, forearm, and arm

Careful breast exam to evaluate for breast mass, cyst, abscess

Check for nipple discharge

Consider measuring each breast in vertical and horizontal planes for comparison with later exams (i.e. 12 to 6 o'clock; 3 to 9 o'clock)

Check for tuberous breast shape (overdeveloped nipple areolar complex with breast tissue limited in vertical and horizontal diameters at the base – looks like a tuberous root plant)

BIBLIOGRAPHY

Cherup LL, Siewers RD, Futrell JW. Breast and pectoral muscle maldevelopment after anterolateral and posterolateral thoracotomies in children. *Ann Thorac Surg* 1986;41:492–7

Jansen DA, Stoetzel RS, Leveque J. Premenarchal athletic injury to the breast bud as the cause for asymmetry: prevention and treatment. *Breast J* 2002;8: 108–11

Templeman C, Hertweck SP. Breast disorders in the pediatric and adolescent patient. *Obstet Gynecol Clin North Am* 2000;27:19–34

7 Breast mass

KEY POINTS

Breast development (thelarche) may be asymmetric and present as a 'breast mass', therefore surgical excision should be reserved for obvious pathologic processes to avoid iatrogenic amastia with excision of the breast bud

Most common masses in this age group are fibroadenomas, followed by fibrocystic changes

Primary breast cancer accounts for less than 1% of all adolescent breast tumors

Malignant breast masses more commonly from metastases of non-breast tissue origin than primary breast cancers (rhabdomyosarcoma, Hodgkin's and non-Hodgkin's lymphoma, neuroblastomas)

Risk of breast cancer as an adult is increased for survivors of childhood malignancy and/or in those treated with thoracic radiation

DIFFERENTIAL DIAGNOSIS

Fibroadenoma (firm, mobile, non-tender)

Fibrocystic changes

Breast cyst

Abscess/mastitis

Intraductal papilloma

Fat necrosis/lipoma

Rare lesions (e.g. hemangiomas, lymphangiomas, lymphoma)

Normal breast tissue

Malignancy

> Primary breast cancer – rare under age 18

> Other malignancies even though rare are more likely than primary breast (e.g. rhabdomyosarcoma, lymphoma, neuroblastoma)

DIAGNOSIS

Ultrasound

   Most useful imaging modality in adolescents

   Can distinguish between solid and cystic masses and help delineate asbscesses (see Breast abscess, Chapter 4)

Self-breast exam (SBE)

   Instruction and use are controversial in adolescents due to low risk of malignancy and high anxiety regarding any mass palpated

   Recommend use in:

   - girls with BRCA1 or BRCA2 beginning at age 18–21 years
   - girls with history of malignancy known to present in the breast (rhabdomyosarcoma, neuroblastoma, lymphoma, leukemia)
   - girls with previous thoracic/chest wall irradiation

Mammography

   Not indicated in patients younger than 25 years

   Increased breast tissue density makes for a less sensitive test

MANAGEMENT

See Figure 7-1

SPECIFIC MASSES

Fibroadenomas:

   Most common breast mass in young girls

   More common in African-Americans

   Rubbery, discrete, non-tender

   Typically 2 to 3 cm at presentation

   Unilateral, upper outer quadrant

   10% regress spontaneously

   Recurrent or multiple in 10–25% of cases

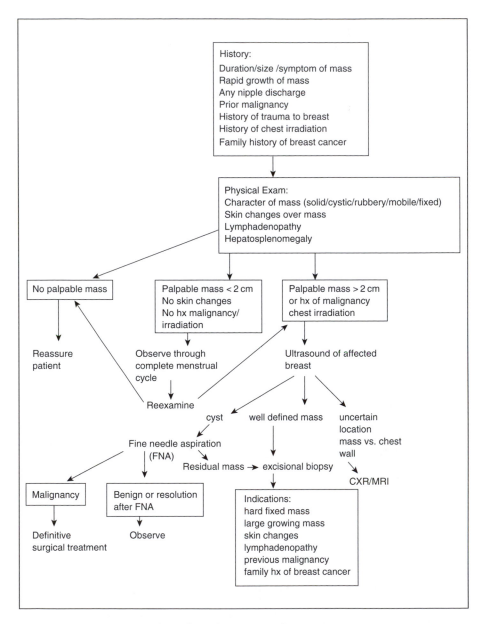

Figure 7-1 Breast mass algorithm: diagnosis and treatment

Giant fibroadenoma

Rapidly increasing asymmetric mass > 5 cm

May have distorted veins over surface

Eventual risk of breast cancer may be slightly higher

Fibrocystic changes:

2nd most common breast abnormality in adolescents

Defined as condition in which mastalgia and breast tenderness are associated with palpable lumps

Symptoms fluctuate with menses

Management options: Oral contraceptives – 70–90% improvement

Oral medroxyprogesterone acetate in luteal phase

Evening primrose oil effective in 44% (1000 mg po tid)

Cysts:

Small cysts (< 2 cm) will often resolve spontaneously

May aspirate larger cysts with fine needle aspiration (see Figure 7-1)

Abscess:

See Breast abscess (Chapter 4)

Cystosarcoma phylloides:

Rare tumor, < 5% in those younger than 20 years

Typically benign, but can be malignant

Malignant potential based on mitotic activity of tumor

Tumor recurrence more common with positive surgical margins/proliferative tumor margins

Slow-growing tumor

Contusion (fat necrosis):

Results from trauma to the breast

Presents as a poorly defined, tender mass

Typically has resolution over several weeks to months

Manage hematomas with analgesics, ice packs and binding of the breast (sports bra or elastic wrap)

BIBLIOGRAPHY

Kaste SC, Hudson MM, Jones DJ, *et al*. Breast masses in women treated for childhood cancer: Incidence and screening guidelines. *Cancer* 1998;82:784–92

Pacinda SJ, Ramzy I. Fine-needle aspiration of breast mass. *J Adolesc Health* 1998;23:3–6

Templeman C, Hertweck SP. Breast disorders in the pediatric and adolescent patient. *Obstet Gynecol Clin* 2000;27:19–34

Weinstein SP, Conant EF, Orel SG, *et al*. Spectrum of ultrasound findings in pediatric and adolescent patients with palpable breast masses. *Radiographics* 2000;20:1613–21

8 Cervical mass

Large differential diagnosis:

Arteriovenous (a-v) malformation, cancer, chancre, chancroid, condyloma, hemangioma, nabothian cyst, polyp, pregnancy

DIAGNOSIS

History

Abnormal bleeding, discharge or odor or may be an incidental finding

Physical examination

In child:

- Use vaginoscopy with/without anesthesia (see Operative Care, Chapter 37)

In adolescent:

- Use appropriate speculum (See Gynecologic examination, Chapter 21). If diagnosis unclear, check pregnancy test. If negative and sexually active perform a Pap test and screen for chlamydia, gonorrhea, and syphilis
- Consider colposcopy to evaluate with biopsy if necessary

MANAGEMENT

Treatment should be diagnosis specific

If purely cystic, lesion can be observed

If diagnosis unclear or mass begins to change, biopsy with anesthesia as needed

If solid and unclear diagnosis needs to be biopsied with anesthesia as needed

If a-v malformation suspected, then use MRI to image. If confirmed or suggestive, consult with vascular surgeon regarding management

> **Do not biopsy without consultation if any suspicion of a vascular abnormality**

9 Clitoromegaly

Clitoral enlargement deserves full attention/thorough evaluation

May be first sign of an endocrine or intersex disorder or an underlying neoplastic process

Clitoral enlargement usually occurs with other signs of virilization like hirsutism, acne and deepening of the voice

May be the presenting sign of neurofibromatosis (typically patients also have café-au-lait macules prior or at time of clitoral enlargement)

DEFINITION

Prepubertal clitoral size:

> Normal: Clitoral glans 3 mm diameter
>
> Abnormal: Clitoral glans > 5 mm or
>
> Clitoral index (glans width × length) > 35 mm

Adolescent/adult clitoral size:

- Normal clitoral glans 2–4 mm wide and 5 mm long
- Total clitoral length (glans and body) 16 mm
- Mean clitoral index (glans width × glans length) 18.5 mm

DIFFERENTIAL DIAGNOSIS

Exposure to androgens

> Maternal drug/androgen exposure in infants
>
> Endogenous (e.g. androgen tumor)
>
> Exogenous (e.g. medications like danazol)

Congenital causes/tumors

    Gonadal dysgenesis

    True hermaphroditism

    Adrenal enzyme deficiency

    Neurofibroma

    Choristoma (aberrant rest or heterotopic tissue)

Clitoral mass

    Epidermal cyst

    Fibroma

    Leiomyoma

    Angiokeratoma

    Pseudolymphoma

    Hemangioma

    Granular cell tumor

    Neurofibroma

Clitoral tumors (rare)

    Rhabdomyosarcoma

    Schwannoma

    Endodermal sinus tumor

    Lymphoma

    Dermoid cyst

DIAGNOSIS

History

Age of patient

- Newborn or infant: work up as for ambiguous genitalia (see Ambiguous genitalia, Chapter 1)
- Children: concern for late onset adrenal enzyme deficiency or exogenous vs endogenous androgen production

Duration of clitoromegaly

Any associated symptoms

- Clitoral pain or irritation
- Acne, facial hair or hirsutism
- Abdominal pain (indicating mass effect)
- Family history
- Neurofibromatosis

Physical examination

Height/weight (plot on growth curves)

Check skin for:

- Café-au-lait spots
- Signs of androgen excess

    Acne

    Hirsutism

    Acanthosis nigricans (darkly pigmented skin of velvety appearance at nape of neck, axilla, waist – indicating insulin resistance, associated with severe polycystic ovarian syndrome (PCOS)/hyperandrogenicity)

Abdomen:

- Look for male escutcheon hair pattern
- Palpate for hepatosplenomegaly, tumors or masses

Pelvic:

- Assess clitoral size (see above definitions)
- Assess external genitalia for normal appearance
- Assess vagina for estrogenization

    (Pale pink with white mucus discharge – estrogenized)

    (Dark red hymen with thin border – atrophic)

- Perform digital bimanual or rectoabdominal bimanual exam to assess adnexa for masses

Laboratory evaluations

Total testosterone level

Dehydroepiandrosterone sulfate (DHEAS) level

7 a.m. 17-hydroxyprogesterone level

Consider karyotype

Imaging

Pelvic ultrasound/imaging studies of ovaries and adrenals if exam unsatisfactory or to confirm findings

If imagining studies negative, may need CT/MRI of clitoris to fully visualize clitoral mass and plan treatment

MANAGEMENT

If clitoromegaly in spectrum of other androgen signs: work up as per hyperandrogenism/PCOS

If isolated clitoromegaly:

If suspect mass effect from tumor – excisional biopsy indicated

If clitoris enlarged with normal laboratory findings – consult with pediatric gynecologist/surgeon/urologist regarding surgical revision

BIBLIOGRAPHY

Levard G, Podevin J, Levillain P, Podevin G. Congenital neoplasm of the clitoris. *J Urol* 1997;157:649

Sane K, Pescovitz OH. The clitoral index: a determination of clitoral size in normal girls and girls with abnormal sexual development. *J Pediatr* 1992; 120:264

Sutphen R, Galan-Gomez E, Kousseff BG. Clitoromegaly in neurofibromatosis. *Am J Med Genet* 1995;55:325–30

Verkauf BS, Von Thron J, O'Brien WF. Clitoral size in normal women. *Obstet Gynecol* 1992;80:41

10 Condyloma acuminatum

Infection caused by human papillomavirus (HPV)

Most common sexually transmitted disease (STD)

Transmission: vertical, innocent and via sexual contact

Incubation period is generally 1–20 months, but latency periods of at least 3 years are known

Most common are non-oncogenic types 6, 11; isolated reports of autoinoculation of type 2 from cutaneous warts; oncogenic types are 16, 18, 31, 33 and others

DIAGNOSIS

Cauliflower, papular lesions that predominate in the anogenital area in prepubertal children; occur anywhere in the genital tract in sexually active adolescents

May present with bleeding, pruritis and pain; can be completely asymptomatic

MANAGEMENT

No data have proven that treatment is preferable to observation for spontaneous regression

If symptomatic, treat:

   If not sexually active, screen carefully for sexual abuse before treatment

   - Document the age when warts were first noted, mode of delivery, any history of warts or HPV in child, family or contacts
   - Physical exam for signs of sexual abuse (see Sexual abuse, Chapter 54)
   - If neither conclusive, forensic interview is recommended at local children's advocacy agency

- HPV typing should not be used to assess sexual abuse; typing methods, even new techniques (i.e. hybrid capture) have cross reactivity as well as false negative results; HPV types have latency and transformation characteristics still not well understood

If sexually active, before treatment perform Pap test and screen for STDs if not done within the last 3 months of the appearance of the condyloma. Encourage careful inspection of partner for visible lesions

Despite successful treatment, can recur. Biopsy if recurs repeatedly and screen for HIV

Treatment

Medical

(Not FDA approved in children)

No treatment is superior; most treatments require more than one dosing

- Imiquimod 5% cream

    Can be very erosive to epithelium particularly in prepubertal child

    Apply test dose with a Q-tip to one lesion very sparingly

    Have patient return in one week and, if no untoward effects, extend the area and frequency of treatment very slowly and check weekly

    Do not treat more frequently than weekly in the prepubertal child and twice weekly in young adolescent

- Intralesional interferon alpha

    Injections are painful and cumbersome with associated fever, myalgia, lethargy and headaches

    Consult with Pediatric Dermatology or Infectious Disease regarding use and dosing

Other less expensive treatments:

- Trichlorocetic acid (TCA) or bichloroacetic acid (BCA) 80–90%

    Apply small amount to the wart with a toothpick

    Lubricate surrounding skin

    Allow to dry to a white coat; may wash off in an hour especially if definitely persistent burning

    Repeat weekly

- Podofilox 0.5% solution or gel

    Patient or parent applies to warts twice daily for 3 days then nothing for 4 days

    Repeat up to 4 cycles

    Treated wart area should be < 10 mm^3

    Limit total volume Podofilox to 0.5 ml/day

    Safety not established in pregnancy would not use in children

- Cimetidine oral tablets or suspension

    40 mg/kg/day in three divided doses

    Usually treat at least 3 months since effects are rarely seen before at least two months

If disease persists without significant change for one month, screen with appropriate serology and tissue specimens for immunodeficiency including human immunodeficiency virus (HIV) and other pathologic causes and check for continued reinfection

Surgical

Only use in recalcitrant symptomatic cases where immune deficiency and other pathologic causes ruled out

CO_2 laser is preferred method

- Advantages: more hemostatic and less tissue damage
- Disadvantages: requires general anesthesia
- *Procedure:*

    Attach laser to the colposcope or microscope with a micromanipulator to best define the dermatologic planes

    Use the superpulse mode at a low wattage – leaves minimal adjuvant tissue damage

    Vaporized debris is frequently wiped away with 3–5% acetic acid-soaked gauze so that the classic white papillations can be observed

- *Postoperatively:*

    Infiltrate operative sites with 0.25% marcaine (plain)

    Prescribe narcotics and NSAIDs (see Operative care, Chapter 37 for dosing)

    Apply ice locally for 48 h as tolerated

    Sitz baths qid followed by airdrying with blowdryer on low setting and silvadene cream applied liberally to area until healed

Void in bathtub or dilute urine with peri-bottle while voiding

Use stool softener (i.e. Colace, Shier US, Inc., Florence, KY) to prevent constipation

If extensive resection, may need hospitalization with Foley catheter overnight

Follow-up

Despite apparent resolution of the lesions, long-term follow-up is indicated because of the known risk of recurrence and unknown risk of eventual development of cervical carcinoma in prepubertal patients with condyloma

In extensive and/or recurrent cases of prepubertal condyloma, frequency of Pap testing is unknown:

* When sexually active: routine yearly vs. 6-month interval
* Non-sexually active: there is no data to assist in this management – may be indicated to initiate Pap testing earlier than age 21

Vaccines are in development in the adult population:

* Primary research has been directed toward a vaccine to stimulate the host response of infected persons against HPV proteins
* In development: a prophylactic vaccine that could be used to prevent infection or at least limit the course of the initial infection

COUNSELING/EDUCATION

Condoms are not 100% effective

Smoking and second-hand smoke inhibit viral clearing

Transmission possible without visible lesions

Male partners with visible lesions in anogenital region should be referred for management

BIBLIOGRAPHY

Centers for Disease Control and Prevention. Sexually transmitted diseases treatment guidelines 2002. *MMWR* 2002;51(No.RR-6)

Gibbs, NF. Anogenital papillomavirus infections in children. *Curr Opin Pediatr* 1998;10:393–7

11 Contraception

KEY POINTS

Refusal to have a pelvic exam at initial visit should not be a barrier to prescribing contraception

Spending time with the adolescent to select a method ensures improved compliance

Method selection should include a hormonal method and a barrier method

If an adolescent's choice is a barrier method only, it should be combined with a second barrier method (i.e. contraceptive cream, foam, jelly or sponge)

Intrauterine devices and diaphragms are not commonly used in the adolescent patient

MANAGEMENT

First visit

Introduction

Explain the need for privacy and confidentiality in the adolescent years

Reassure the parents that the provider will share as much as possible but that certain information about school, friends, drugs, and sexuality needs to remain confidential unless the information indicates a life-threatening situation

When the adolescent requests that her sexual activity be kept confidential, the clinician and the young woman need to agree in private how they will explain the planned therapy to the parent, i.e. dysmenorrhea or irregular menses

Discuss method of payment for the visit, laboratory tests and medications. Patients may need to be referred to Planned Parenthood or the Health Department if insurance cannot be billed in a confidential manner

Involvement of the partner should be encouraged

History

Obtain a complete family and medical history

Obtain review of systems to identify issues of weight gain, headaches, acne, breast tenderness, dysmenorrhea, irregular menses and nausea/vomiting

Assess psychosocial factors that will help to determine compliance and hence effectiveness. Multiple partners, low self esteem and feelings of hopelessness are associated with poor compliance. Strong academic performance and established career goals are associated with successful use of contraception

See Figure 21-14, the self-administered confidential adolescent questionnaire in Gynecologic examination (Chapter 21).

Physical examination

Check blood pressure, height and weight

Examination of the breast, heart, thyroid, abdomen and extremities

Pelvic examination should be performed; with the proper pre-examination instruction, demonstration and support staff most sexually active teens will feel comfortable undergoing a pelvic exam at their first visit; inability to obtain a pelvic exam should not be a barrier to contraception

Laboratory Tests

Pap test, *Neisseria gonorrhoeae*, *Chlamydia trachomatis*, syphilis and HIV screening (if indicated), and hepatitis B screen if not immunized (immunization should be encouraged for those non-immune)

Pregnancy test and urinalysis if warranted by history

Thrombophilia work-up if a significant family history of early venous thromboembolic disease (less than age 55): Screen for Factor V Leiden and prothrombin mutation, antithrombin III, fasting homocysteine, protein C, protein S levels

Lipid panel, fasting if a significant family history (either parent) of lipid disorder

Selection of a method

Discuss all available hormonal methods including emergency contraception (ECP)

Emphasize the importance of using a hormonal contraceptive and a barrier

Discuss previous methods and any issues with that method

Discuss myths of contraception

> Weight gain: yes on Depo-Provera; uncommon on combined oral contraceptives (COCs)
>
> Acne: improved on COCs
>
> Infertility: no causal effects
>
> Cancer: no causal effects; may protect against uterine and ovarian
>
> Promotes sexual debut: no causal effects
>
> Bone loss: possible with Depo-Provera (see Osteoporosis, Chapter 38); not with COCs
>
> Dysmenorrhea: yes, all can help
>
> Ovarian cysts: yes, all can help
>
> Good time to discuss substance use and cessation, particularly tobacco

Contraindication to combination (estrogen and progestin) contraceptives

> Thrombophlebitis or thromboembolic disorders – past or present
>
> Cerebral vascular/coronary artery disease
>
> Known or suspected carcinoma of the breast
>
> Carcinoma of the endometrium
>
> Undiagnosed abnormal genital bleeding
>
> Cholestatic jaundice of pregnancy or with previous contraceptive use
>
> Hepatic disease, adenomas or carcinomas
>
> Sickle cell disease
>
> Breastfeeding

Precautions to combination contraceptives

> Third generation progestins: presently, controversy over potential increased venous thromboembolism (VTE) in adults
>
> Migraine headaches with focal neurologic symptoms

Seizures controlled by medication

Recent mononucleosis

Cardiac valvular disease

Pancreatitis

Collagen vascular disease

Gallbladder disease

Inflammatory bowel disease

Tobacco smoking: increased thrombosis from synergism with estrogen

Controlled hypertension

Precautions to progestin only contraceptives

Obesity

Potential for abnormal bone density (low body mass index, chronic steroid use, non-weight bearing)

Known or suspected pregnancy

Bleeding disorder

Hair loss

Depression

SPECIFIC CONTRACEPTIVE METHOD INSTRUCTION

ESTROGEN AND PROGESTIN COMBINATION CONTRACEPTIVES

Combined estrogen–progestin oral contraceptive pills

Start:

1st day of menses or after first trimester abortion *or*

1st Sunday after period begins *or*

Today if you're sure you're not pregnant (more likely to be compliant) *or*

At least two weeks or more postpartum if not breastfeeding; 6 weeks postpartum if breastfeeding

Effective:

After 1 package

After 7 continuous days of pills, if you have missed two or less pills

Ineffective:

On first package, if you have missed one or more pills

With diarrhea or vomiting

With drugs that change liver function or decrease the body's ability to absorb hormones, i.e. rifampin, Dilantin (Parke-Davis, Morris Plains, NJ), carbamazepine, tetracycline, ampicillin

Follow up 6 weeks after starting:

Check blood pressure and weight

Check urine human chorionic gonadotropin (hCG)

Check untoward side effects, i.e. ACHES (Abdominal or extremity pain, Chest pain, Headache, Eye problems, Shortness of breath or leg Swelling), nausea, missed pills, condom use

It is helpful to have patient bring the present pill package with them to verify the number of missed pills and correlate with the pills in the pack; ensure that they are inserting refills correctly into the container

May be helpful to review menstrual calendar to assess for breakthrough bleeding

Missed pill regime:

Miss one pill, take it as soon as you remember or the next day. Use additional contraception for 7 days. Expect breakthrough bleeding.

Miss two pills, double up for two days in a row. Use additional contraception for 7 days. Expect some nausea (try to space out each pill slightly) and breakthrough bleeding

Miss three pills or more, put the pack aside as an extra, wait for some bleeding and begin a new pill pack the Sunday after bleeding occurred

Combination oral contraceptive pill types and doses

See Table 11-1

Monthly injection – medroxyprogesterone acetate/estradiol cypionate (Lunelle®, Pharmacia & Upjohn, Peapack, NJ)

Start:

First 5 days of a normal menses or after a first trimester abortion; 4 weeks postpartum, if not breastfeeding; 6 weeks postpartum, if breastfeeding

Effective:

Immediately; must be repeated monthly (up to 33 days)

Ineffective:

When used in conjunction with aminoglutethimide (Cytadren®, Novartis Consumer Health, Summit, NJ)

Follow-up:

As with COCs

Transdermal patch – norelgestromin/ethinyl estradiol (OrthoEvra®, Ortho-McNeil Pharmaceutical Inc., Raritan, NJ)

Start:

First day of menses or on the day of a first trimester abortion or the first Sunday after; no earlier than four weeks postpartum, if not breastfeeding; 6 weeks postpartum, if breastfeeding

Effective:

It takes 2 days to achieve therapeutic levels of hormones after application of the patch. A new patch is applied every 7 days for 3 weeks followed by a patch-free fourth week

Ineffective:

Body weight >198 lbs (90 kg) and COC restrictions

Follow-up:

As with COCs

Vaginal ring – etonogestrel/ethinyl estradiol (NuvaRing®, Organon, Inc., West Orange, NJ)

Start:

Within 5 days after the beginning of a period

Effective:

7 days after insertion as long as it has not been dislodged for more than 3 hours; must be left in for 3 weeks, then out for 1 week and new one reinserted

Ineffective:

As with COCs

Follow-up:

As with COCs

Table 11-1   Oral contraceptive pill types and doses*

Progestin only:	Micronor (Ortho)	progestin only	Norethindrone = 0.35 mg
	Nor-QD (Watson)	progestin only	Norethindrone = 0.35 mg
	Ovrette (Wyeth-Ayerst)	progestin only	Norgestrel = 0.075 mg
20 micrograms:	Alesse (Wyeth-Ayerst)	EE = 20 μg	Levonorgestrel = 0.1 mg
	LevLite (Berlex)	EE = 20 μg	Levonorgestrel = 0.1 mg
	Loestrin FE 1/20 (Parke-Davis)	EE = 20 μg/ 75 mg ferrous fumarate (7d)	Norethindrone = 1 mg
	Mircette (Organon)	EE = 20 μg	Desogestrel = 0.15 mg
30 micrograms:	Desogen Tablets (Organon)	EE = 30 μg	Desogestrel = 0.15 mg
	LevLen (Berlex)	EE = 30 μg	Levonorgestrel = 0.15 mg
	Levora (Watson)	EE = 30 μg	Levonorgestrel = 0.15 mg
	Loestrin 21 1.5/30 (Parke-Davis)	EE = 30 μg	Norethindrone = 1.5 mg
	Lo/Ovral Tablets (Wyeth-Ayerst)	EE = 30 μg	Norgestrel = 0.30 mg
	Lo/Ovral-28 Tablets	EE = 30 μg	Norgestrel = 0.30 mg
	Nordette-21 Tablets	EE = 30 μg	Levonorgestrel = 0.15 mg
	Nordette-28 Tablets (Wyeth-Ayerst)	EE = 30 μg	Levonorgestrel = 0.15 mg
	Ortho-Cept 21 Tablets (Ortho)	EE = 30 μg	Desogestrel = 0.15 mg
	Ortho-Cept 28 Tablets	EE = 30 μg	Desogestrel = 0.15 mg
	Yasmin Tablets (Berlex)	EE = 30 μg	Drospirenone = 3.0 mg
35 micrograms:	Brevicon 21-day (Roche)	EE = 35 μg	Norethindrone = 0.5 mg
	Brevicon 28-day	EE = 35 μg	Norethindrone = 0.5 mg
	Demulen 1/35-21 (Searle)	EE = 35 μg	Ethynodiol =1 mg
	Demulen 1/35-28	EE = 35 μg	Ethynodiol = 1 mg
	Jenest 28 (Organon)	EE = 35 μg	Norethindrone = 0.5/1 mg
	Modicon 21 Tablets (Ortho)	EE = 35 μg	Norethindrone = 0.5 mg
	Modicon 28 Tablets	EE = 35 μg	Norethindrone = 0.5 mg
	Necon 1/35 28 (Watson)	EE = 35 μg	Norethindrone = 1 mg
	Norethin 1/35E-28 (Searle)	EE = 35 μg	Norethindrone = 1 mg
	Norinyl 1+35 21-day (Roche)	EE = 35 μg	Norethindrone = 1 mg
	Norinyl 1+35 28-day	EE = 35 μg	Norethindrone = 1 mg
	Ortho-Cyclen 21 Tablets (Ortho)	EE = 35 μg	Norgestimate = 0.25 mg
	Ortho-Cyclen 28 Tablets	EE = 35 μg	Norgestimate = 0.25 mg
	Ortho-Novum 1/35-21	EE = 35 μg	Norethindrone = 1 mg
	Ortho-Novum 1/35-28	EE = 35 μg	Norethindrone = 1 mg

(Continued)

Table 11-1 (Continued)

	Ortho-Novum 7/7/7-21	EE = 35 µg	Norethindrone = 0.5/0.75/1 mg
	Ortho-Novum 7/7/7-28	EE = 35 µg	Norethindrone = 0.5/0.75/1 mg
	Ortho-Novum 10/11-21	EE = 35 µg	Norethindrone = 0.5/1 mg
	Ortho-Novum 10/11-28	EE = 35 µg	Norethindrone = 0.5/1 mg
	Ortho Tri-Cyclen 21	EE = 35 µg	Norgestimate = 0.18/ 0.215/0.25 mg
	Ortho Tri-Cyclen 28	EE = 35 µg	Norgestimate = 0.18/ 0.215/0.25 mg
	Ovcon 35-21 (Bristol-Myers Squibb)	EE = 35 µg	Norethindrone = 0.4 mg
	Ovcon 35-28	EE = 35 µg	Norethindrone = 0.4 mg
	Tri-Norinyl 21-Day Tablets (Roche)	EE = 35 µg	Norethindrone = 0.5 mg
	Tri-Norinyl 28-Day Tablets	EE = 35 µg	Norethindrone = 0.5 mg
	Zovia 1/35-28 (Watson)	EE = 35 µg	Ethynodiol diacetate = 1 mg
50 micrograms:	Demulen 1/50-21	EE = 50 µg	Ethynodiol = 1 mg
	Demulen 1/50-28	EE = 50 µg	Ethynodiol = 1 mg
	Norinyl 1+50 21-day (Roche)	EE = 50 µg	Norethindrone = 1 mg
	Norinyl 1+50 28-day	EE = 50 µg	Norethindrone = 1 mg
	Ortho-Novum 1/50-21 (Ortho)	EE = 50 µg	Norethindrone = 1 mg
	Ortho-Novum 1/50-28	EE = 50 µg	Norethindrone = 1 mg
	Ovcon 50-28	EE = 50 µg	Norethindrone = 1 mg
	Ovral Tablets (Wyeth-Ayerst)	EE = 50 µg	Norgestrel = 0.5 mg
	Ovral-28 Tablets	EE = 50 µg	Norgestrel = 0.5 mg
	Zovia 1/50E-21 (Watson)	EE = 50 µg	Ethynodiol diacetate = 1 mg
Multiphasics:	Estrostep FE (Parke-Davis)	EE = 20/30/ 35 µg/75 mg ferrous fumarate(7d)	Norethindrone =1 mg
	Ortho Tri Cyclen Lo (Ortho-McNeil)	EE = 25 µg	Norgestimate = 180 µg/ 215 µg/250 µg
	Estrostep 21	EE = 20/30/35 µg	Norethindrone =1 mg
	Tri LevLen (Berlex)	EE = 30/40/30 µg	Levonorgestrel = 0.050/0.075/0.125 mg
	Triphasil-21 Tablets (Wyeth-Ayerst)	EE = 30/40/30 µg	Levonorgestrel = 0.050/0.075/0.125 mg
	Triphasil-28 Tablets	EE = 30/40/30 µg	Levonorgestrel = 0.050/ 0.075/0.125 mg

Currently available in the United States

EE, ethinyl estradiol
Revised with permission from: Association of Reproductive Health Professionals, Washington, DC. www.ARHP.org

PROGESTIN ONLY CONTRACEPTIVES

Depot medroxyprogesterone acetate (Depo-Provera®, Pharmacia & Upjohn, Peapack, NJ)

Start:

> First 5 days of a normal menstrual cycle or after first trimester abortion; first 5 days postpartum if not breastfeeding; 6th week postpartum if solely breastfeeding; after abstaining from sexual activity for 14 days followed by a negative quantitative hCG

Effective:

> Immediately except for the last category (abstaining for 14 days) then not effective for 21 days

> Must be repeated up to every 13 weeks

Ineffective:

> More than 13 weeks since the last shot

> With use of medication: aminoglutethimide (Cytadren®)

Follow-up:

> Yearly annual gynecologic exam (see Gynecologic examination, Chapter 21)

> If amenorrhea > 1 year consider evaluation of bone density (see Osteoporosis, Chapter 28)

Progestin only pill – minipill

See Table 11-1 for types and doses

Start:

> First day of menses or first Sunday after menses or the day of a first trimester abortion

Effective:

> After one week without missed pills; pills have to be taken every day; less effective than COCs and Depo-Provera®

Ineffective:

> Medication: hepatic enzyme inducing drugs
> * Anticonvulsants: phenytoin, carbamazapine, barbituates
> * Antituberculosis: rifampin

Follow-up:

> Same as Depo-Provera®

> If amenorrhea for more than two packages and sexually active should perform pregnancy test

BARRIER/NON-HORMONAL METHODS

Condoms (male, female, latex, non-latex)

Should demonstrate proper usage with patient

Should give a pamphlet to share with partner about proper use and STDs

Provide samples

BIBLIOGRAPHY

Blum RW. Sexual health contraceptive needs of adolescents with chronic conditions. *Arch Pediatr Adolesc Med* 1997;151:290–6

Hatcher RA, Trussell J, Stewart F, *et al. Contraceptive Technology*, 17th edn. New York: Ardent Media, 1998

Hatcher RA, Nelson AL, Zieman M, *et al.* A *Pocket Guide to Managing Contraception*: 2002–2003. Tiger, GA: Bridging the Gap Foundation, 2002

12 Depression

Depression is twice as likely to develop in teenage girls than boys during adolescence

40–70% of depressed children and adolescents have comorbid psychiatric disorders

Risk factors

Family history of depression in first-degree relatives

Prior depressive episodes

Attention deficit hyperactivity disorder (ADHD)

Family dysfunction

Peer problems

Academic difficulties

Negative mode of interpreting events and coping with stress

Comorbidity

Most frequent comorbidities:

- Substance abuse
- Anxiety disorders
- Disruptive behaviors (e.g. ADHD)
- Eating disorders
- Learning disorders

DIAGNOSIS

Major depressive disorder (DSM–IV criteria)

- Either depressed mood or loss in interest or pleasure most of the day, nearly every day for a 2-week period

- May manifest as irritability, boredom vs sadness or depression
- In addition at least 4 of the following must be present:

  Significant weight loss

  Insomnia or hypersomnia

  Psychomotor agitation or retardation

  Fatigue or loss of energy

  Feelings of worthlessness or inappropriate guilt

  Diminished ability to think

  Recurrent thoughts of death/suicide

Differential diagnosis

Mood disorder related to medical condition (e.g. hypothyroidism, mononucleosis)

Substance-induced mood disorder (e.g. drug abuse)

Bereavement

Adjustment disorder

Bipolar disorder

History

Ask in nonstigmatizing way:

- 'Everyone I know gets sad sometimes, what kind of things make you sad?'
- 'On a scale of 1 to 10 how annoyed have you been lately?'

Use standardized instrument:

- Beck Depression Inventory (BDI) in adolescents
- Pediatric Symptom Checklist for parents of children ages 6 to 12 years

Do comprehensive initial assessment for comorbid conditions as above

- Evaluate in context of precipitants, stressors, academic, social and family function

Ask about suicidal ideation

MANAGEMENT

If suicidal, immediate psychiatric intervention necessary

If not suicidal but major depression diagnosis:

> Educate patient's parent, put symptoms into context to permit psychotherapy to occur (e.g. 'You've been experiencing considerable fatigue that has been immobilizing; it is very common to feel discouraged, annoyed or even depressed when faced with this stress day in and day out.')
>
> Refer to psychiatry/psychology

Treatment with medication

> Cochrane Database information regarding use of tricyclic antidepressants in children and adolescents found that they are not useful in treating depression in pre-pubertal children

> There is marginal evidence to support their use in adolescents

> There is also limited evidence-based information about the use of selective serotonin reuptake inhibitors (SSRIs) in the pediatric and adolescent population

> Recommend consultation with a child psychiatrist or psychopharmacologist prior to prescribing medication

BIBLIOGRAPHY

Beasley PJ, Beardslee WR. Depression in the adolescent patient. *Adolesc Med State of the Art Rev* 1998;9:351–62

Beck AT, Ward CH, Mendelson M, *et al*. An inventory for measuring depression. *Arch Gen Psychiatry* 1961;4:561

Bobin L. Depression in adolescents: Epidemiology, clinical manifestations and diagnosis. *UptoDate* 2002

Hazell P, O'Connell D, Heathcote D, *et al*. Tricyclic drugs for depression in children and adolescents. *The Cochrane Library* 2002;4

Jellinek MS, Murphy JM, Robinson J, *et al*. Pediatric symptom checklist: screening school-age children for psychosocial dysfunction. *J Pediatr* 1988;112:201–9

13 Dysfunctional uterine bleeding (DUB)

Usually due to anovulatory cycles

Important to consider possibility of coagulation defect or sexually transmitted diseases (STDs) (e.g. chlamydia) as other common causes

DEFINITION

Excessive, prolonged or irregular bleeding from the endometrium unrelated to anatomic lesions of the uterus

Variation in frequency:

- Polymenorrhea: frequent regular or irregular bleeding at < 21 day intervals

- Oligomenorrhea: infrequent irregular bleeding at > 35 day intervals

- Irregular menses: bleeding at varying intervals >21 days but < 45 days

Variation in amount and duration:

Metrorrhagia: intermenstrual irregular bleeding between regular periods

Menorrhagia: excessive amount and increased duration of uterine bleeding occurring regularly

Menometrorrhagia: frequent irregular, excessive and prolonged episodes of uterine bleeding > 7 days in duration

DIFFERENTIAL DIAGNOSIS

- Anovulation
    - Immaturity of hypothalamic–pituitary–ovarian axis
    - Hypothalamic dysfunction
    - Polycystic ovarian syndrome
- Pregnancy-related conditions
    - Missed, threatened or spontaneous abortion
    - Retained products after elective abortion
- Coagulation disorders
    - Von Willebrand's disease
    - Platelet aggregation defect
    - Idiopathic thrombocytopenic purpura
- Anatomic
    - Mullerian anomalies (e.g. uterine didelphys with hemi-obstructed vagina and perforation)
- Chronic or systemic diseases
    - Diabetes mellitus
    - Hepatic dysfunction
    - Renal dysfunction
    - Thyroid dysfunction
- Trauma
    - Accidental injury
    - Coital trauma
    - Sexual abuse
    - Vaginal foreign body
- Lower reproductive tract infections
    - *Chlamydia trachomatis*
    - Pelvic inflammatory disease
- Endocrine disorders
    - Functional ovarian hyperandrogenism
    - Adrenal excess androgen production
    - Thyroid disorders
    - Hyperprolactinemia

- Eating disorders
    Anorexia, bulimia
- Neoplasms
    Vaginal/cervical tumors

    Endometrial hyperplasia

    Hemangiomas

    Leiomyoma (rare in adolescents)

    Hormonally active ovarian tumors (granulosa cell tumor)
- Medication/drug use
    Exogenous hormone use

DIAGNOSIS

History

- Menstrual history:
    Date/age of menarche (see Menstruation, Chapter 31)

    Frequency of menstrual cycles

    Date/length of most recent menses

    Amount of pads/tampons per day used (soaking through one pad/hour is excessive)
- Evaluate for coagulation defects:
    History of epistaxis, gingival bleeding

    History of peri- or post-operative bleeding

    Family history of coagulation problems
- Medications including
    Oral contraceptives/centrally acting medications
- Confidential sexual history:
    Chlamydial infection can cause DUB
- Related health issues:
    Weight change

    Nutrition history

    Exercise history (excessive exercise)

    Eating disorders/issues

Physical examination

- Vital signs:

    Pulse, blood pressure (look for signs of anemia, check for orthostasis)

    Height, weight, body mass index (extremes in weight associated with anovulation)

- General:

    Look for signs of androgen excess:

    Hirsutism/acne/acanthosis nigricans

- Thyroid:

    Palpate for enlargement

- Breast:

    Assess pubertal development

    Tanner stage

- Abdomen:

    Assess for tenderness/mass

- Pelvic: (use Huffman speculum)

    Assess for anatomic/traumatic source of bleeding

    Rule out foreign body

    Rule out reproductive tract laceration

    Assess cervix

    Rule out inflammation/lesion

    Do STD testing for chlamydia/gonorrhea if patient sexually active

    Assess uterine/adnexal size

    Rule out pregnancy/ovarian mass

- Pelvic ultrasound

    If unsure of adequacy of bimanual exam

    or

    Adnexal mass noted on exam

    or

    If bleeding persistent despite medical management (rule out mullerian anomaly, i.e. perforated hemivagina with uterine didelphys)

Laboratory evaluation

- Baseline:

    Complete blood count with platelet count

    Blood smear

    Pregnancy test

- Recurrent/severe bleeding or menarcheal onset:

    Coagulation profile

    > Von Willebrand factor antigen level*

    > Ristocetin cofactor activity level*

    > Factor VIII coagulant antigen

    > Platelet aggregation studies

    Thyroid stimulating hormone level

    Prothrombin time/partial thromboplastin time (PT/PTT)

    *Note: Draw von Willebrand levels during the menstrual cycle when the estradiol levels are lowest. Von Willebrand factor increases with increasing estrogen levels

- Chronic anovulation/irregular bleeding:

    Follicle stimulating hormone level

    Prolactin level

- DUB with hirsutism:

    Total testosterone

    Dehydroepiandrosterone sulfate level

    7 a.m. 17-hydroxyprogesterone level

MANAGEMENT

- Based on: Presenting signs/symptoms

    Examination findings/laboratory findings

    Presence/absence/severity of anemia

    DUB is a diagnosis of exclusion; if evaluation negative for other causes treat based on below:

Treatment

- Mild cases (bleeding 20–60 day intervals, hemoglobin >11 g/dl)

  Reassurance

  Educate how to keep menstrual calendar

  Iron supplementation

  OCP for contraceptive needs

  Reevaluate in 3 months

- Moderate cases (hemoglobin 9–11 g/dl)

  Educate regarding maintenance of menstrual calendar

  Rule out coagulopathy/treat STD if suspected or detected

  Iron supplementation

  If actively bleeding:

  OCP taper:

  LoOvral® (30 µg ethinyl estradiol/ 0.3 mg norgestrel)

  1 pill every 6 hours × 2 days then

  1 pill every 8 hours × 2 days then

  1 pill every 12 hours × 2 days then

  1 pill daily for 3 days then

  Open new pack Lo-Ovral take daily

  Cycle monthly until hemoglobin normal

  May need antiemetic pre-OCP dose to prevent nausea

  If not actively bleeding:

  Cyclic progestin therapy

  Medroxyprogesterone 10 mg daily × 12 days/month

  or

  Norethindrone acetate 5–10 mg orally daily for 10–14 days a month

  Monophasic low-dose oral contraceptive pill

  Prefer 35 µg ethinyl estradiol/1 mg norgestimate or 30 µg ethinyl estradiol/0.3 mg norgestrel

  Reevaluate in 3 cycles

- Severe cases (hemoglobin < 9 g/dl)

    Acute/anovulatory bleeding (stable patient):

    Rule out coagulopathy

    Ovral (50 µg ethinyl estradiol / 0.5 mg norgestrel)

    Take one pill every 6 hours until bleeding stops

    With menstrual cessation: taper pills

    One pill every 8 hours × 2 days

    Then one pill every 12 hours × 2 days

    Then one pill every day to complete 30 days

    May need antiemetic pre-OCP dose to prevent nausea

    Iron supplementation

    Cycle on OCP for 6 months

    Reevaluation in 4–6 weeks

Acute hemorrhage (hypotension; hemoglobin < 8 g/dl)

    Admit to hospital

    Fluid resuscitation

    Rule out coagulopathy, STD

        Consider hematology consult

    Consider transfusion if symptomatic

        Consider monitoring EKG and oxygen saturation until hemodynamically stable

        Consider use of monitored ICU bed if patient hemodynamically unstable

    Hormonal hemostasis:

    Monophasic 50 µg ethinyl estradiol/ 0.5 mg norgestrel (prefer to use Ovral vs generics due to possible break through bleeding)

        One pill every 6 hours until bleeding stops

        Then one pill every 8 hours for 2 days

        Then one pill every 12 hours for 2 days

        Then one pill every day to complete 30 days

        Allow menses to occur and Sunday start new pack OCPs

Use antiemetic with each dose after the first

If emesis a problem, consider

Conjugated estrogen 25 mg IV every 4–6 hours until bleeding stops

Then Ovral taper as above

If bleeding has not stopped in 48 hours, consider examination under anesthesia, with hysteroscopy

D&C as last resort

Note: Patients with von Willebrand's disease or platelet functional defects (PFD) may respond to use of intranasal Desmopressin acetate (Aventis Pharmaceutical) (DDAVP) which augments hemostasis by increasing levels of circulating von Willebrand factor and factor VIII as well as by nonspecifically shortening the bleeding time in patients with PFD

BIBLIOGRAPHY

Beven JA, Maloney KW, Hillery CA, *et al*. Bleeding disorders: A common cause of menorrhagia in adolescents. *J Pediatr* 2001;138:856–61

Blythe MJ. Common menstrual problems of adolescence. *Adolesc Med: State of the Art Rev* 1997;8:87–109

Bravender T, Emans SJ. Menstrual disorders: Dysfunctional uterine bleeding. *Pediatr Clin North Am* 1999;46:545–53

14 Dysmenorrhea

DEFINITION

Pain during menses; can have associated nausea, vomiting and diarrhea

Primary: painful menstruation in the absence of specific pathologic conditions; more likely if presents later in the menstrual years

Secondary: painful menstruation in the presence of pathologic conditions of the pelvic organs, such as endometriosis, salpingitis, obstipation, adhesions, or congenital anomalies of the mullerian system; more likely if presents early in the menstrual years particularly at the beginning

DIAGNOSIS

History

Age at menarche; menstrual pattern

Description of menstrual pain and other associated symptoms

Response to analgesic medication

Sexual activity; sexual abuse history

Contraceptive and condom use

History of sexually transmitted diseases

History of vaginal discharge

School performance and school absenteeism associated with menstrual problems

Family (particularly mother's) history of menstrual problems

Brief physical examination

Check height, weight, blood pressure

Thyroid and breast exam

Heart and lung exam

Careful abdominal exam

Musculoskeletal exam to elicit any trigger points (see Pelvic pain, Chapter 44)

Vaginal speculum and bimanual exam optional given age; can offer rectoabdominal instead of vaginal exam; can offer ultrasound exam

Rule out other causes

Pathologic lesions, i.e. obstructive mullerian anomaly, obstipation, endometriosis, adhesions, infection

Anovulation

MANAGEMENT

Careful age appropriate explanation of the etiology:

- Prostaglandin build-up leads to vigorous contractions of the uterus
- Changes in behavior and medications can block this build-up

Encourage exercise modifications, i.e. increasing amount of weight bearing exercise one week before menses, well-balanced meals, and stress reduction; if no improvement add non-steroidal antiinflammatory drugs (NSAIDs)

Treatment

NSAIDs

Watch for gastric upset, take with small food portions

Should try to do a loading regimen 48 h before the dysmenorrhea and continue at regular dose until menses ceases

Very individual response, if one type does not work try another

Use cautiously in renal and hepatic insufficiency

Types of NSAIDs:

- Naproxen sodium and ibuprofen (in doses greater than 200 mg) are available as prescription medication (brand names may be more effective than generics)
- Ibuprofen 200–800 mg every 6 to 8 h
- Naproxen sodium 440–550 mg initially, followed by 220–275 mg every 8 h (depending on formulation)
- Mefenamic acid 500 mg initially, followed by 250 mg every 6 h
- Rofecoxib 50 mg every day

- (use cautiously in renal and hepatic insufficiency)
- Not evaluated for safety/efficacy in patients < 18 years

Thermacare®

Use of topical heat such as the ThermaCare® wrap (Procter & Gamble, Cincinnati, OH) has a synergistic effect when used with NSAIDs such as ibuprofen

When NSAIDs fail try hormonal treatment

Combination oral contraceptive pills (COCs) – prefer monophasic, brand name preparations; if no improvement:

Depo-Provera® (Pharmacia & Upjohn, Peapack, NJ) or LupronDepot® (TAP, Lake Forest, IL) to induce amenorrhea; (See Endometriosis (Chapter 18) for dosing instructions; see Osteoporosis, Chapter 38)

When hormones fail

Laparoscopy to rule out endometriosis and/or structural abnormality and/or other cause

BIBLIOGRAPHY

Schroeder B, Sanfilippo JS. Dysmenorrhea and pelvic pain in adolescents. *Pediatr Clin North Am* 1999;46:555–71

15 Eating disorders

DSM–IV DEFINITIONS

Anorexia nervosa

Refusal to maintain weight within a normal range for height and age (more than 15% below ideal body weight)

Intense fear of becoming fat or gaining weight

Disturbed body image such that body image is main measure of self-worth with denial of seriousness of illness

Amenorrhea greater than 3 cycles

Bulimia nervosa

Recurrent episodes of binge eating

> Eating a substantially larger amount of food in a discrete period of time than would be eaten by most people

> A sense of lack of control over eating during the binge

Inappropriate compensatory behaviors to prevent weight gain (e.g. self-induced vomiting, laxative use, fasting, excessive exercise)

Frequency: binges/behaviors occur on average twice/week for at least 3 months

Inappropriate self-evaluation overly influenced by body shape or weight

DIAGNOSIS

History

Patients may present with related problems and/or try to conceal or deny an eating disorder

Look for clues:

Anorexia	Bulimia
Constipation	Mouth sores
Bloating	Dental caries
Early satiety from delayed gastric emptying	Heartburn
Dry skin/cold intolerance	Chest pain
Blue hands/feet	Muscle cramps
Weakness/fatigue	Weakness
Scalp hair loss	Bloody diarrhea (with laxative abuse)
Primary or secondary amenorrhea	Amenorrhea or oligomenorrhea
Easy bruising	Easy bruising

Ask:

How does the patient feel about her body?

- Do you have any 'trouble spots' like the stomach or thighs?
- How hard do you struggle to lose or maintain weight?
- What is the most you ever weighed? And the least? And when did each of those weights occur?
- How much would you like to weigh?

Ask about related behaviors

- What do you do to control your weight?
- Exercise? What kind? How often? How do you feel if you miss a workout?
- Diets/medications/vomiting?

    Have you ever tried diets/medications or vomiting to control your weight?

    Determine frequency, duration of use and day of last use

    Are there any triggers that influence that choice? (such as consuming a certain amount of food or stress)
- Food habits

    Take a 24-hour recall diet history by recounting everything eaten in the past day

    Ask how many bites or what size portions
- Binges

    Ask if the patient ever binges on food

How much and what kind of foods are consumed

Are there any triggers for binging? (time of day, boredom, anger, etc.)

Menstrual history

- Age at menarche, regularity of menses and 1st day of the last two menstrual cycles
- If amenorrheic, what did she weigh during the last period?

Social history

- Ask about school performance (typically anorexics are good students)
- Ask about how the family functions
- Any life stressors in family (divorce, death)
- Any personal or family history of depression
- Any history of sexual abuse

Assess risk taking behaviors

- Sexual activity, tobacco, alcohol or drug use

Physical examination

Height, weight

- May help to look at growth curves if available from pediatrician/family physician
- Consider weighing patient in hospital gown to avoid increase in weight from clothing
- Calculate body mass index (see Obesity, Chapter 35); if < 5th percentile, assess for anorexia

Pulse, blood pressure (both supine and standing)

- Look for bradycardia/hypotension

Body temperature

- Look for hypothermia

Skin/extremity evaluation

- Look for dryness/bruising/lanugo/sagging skin
- Look for calluses in one or more knuckles (Russell's sign)

  Evidence of trauma from scraping teeth with finger-induced vomiting

ENT

- Look for mouth sores, dental erosions on lingual surface of incisors from repeated contact with gastric acid seen with repeated emesis
- Look for parotid gland swelling secondary to vomiting

Breast exam

- Look for atrophy

Cardiac evaluation

- Look for bradycardia/arrhythmia or cardiac murmur due to floppy mitral valve (prolapse)

Abdomen

- Look for scaphoid appearance, pathology as cause of weight loss/vomiting
- Evaluate for mass; rule out malignancy

Pelvic exam

- Assess for vaginal atrophy/dryness due to hypoestrogenization
- Evaluate for pelvic mass/malignancy
- In some cases due to atrophy with hypoestrogenic state a pelvic exam cannot be completed with comfort, therefore substitute with ultrasound

Neurological assessment

- Look for signs of brain tumor (cause for weight loss/vomiting)

Laboratory evaluation

Complete blood count (CBC): rule out anemia, hemoglobin could be high if dehydrated, leukopenia

Erythrocyte sedimentation rate (ESR): rule out chronic illness – should be low with eating disorder

Electrolytes: hypokalemia may indicate vomiting

Calcium, magnesium, phosphorus, blood urea nitrogen (BUN), creatinine

Human chorionic gonadotropin (hCG) if oligomenorrheic or amenorrheic

Urinalysis: assess specific gravity; if low consider water loading to falsely elevate weight

Follicle stimulating hormone (FSH), thyroid stimulating hormone (TSH), prolactin: rule out central causes of oligomenorrhea or amenorrhea

Cholesterol: could be falsely elevated due to low triiodothyronine (T3) levels that inhibit cholesterol breakdown; cholesterol binding globulin may also be low and intrahepatic cholesterol may leak into peripheral circulation

Thyroid function tests: may reveal euthyroid sick syndrome with decreased peripheral conversion of thyroxine (T4) to T3 and high or high normal reverse T3 – an adaptation to starvation to reduce metabolic rate

Bone density evaluation if primary amenorrhea or secondary amenorrhea greater than one year

EKG: do if heart rate (HR) < 50 bpm

- Look for sinus bradycardia
- Sinus tachycardia
- Low voltage P waves and QRS complexes
- Rightward QRS axis
- Non-specific T wave abnormalities
- U waves
- ST segment depression
- Conduction abnormalities
- QT interval prolongation

TREATMENT

Hospitalization

Hospitalize if:

- Severe malnutrition (weight < 75% ideal body weight (IBW))
- Dehydration
- Electrolyte disturbances (hypokalemia, hypophosphatemia)
- EKG abnormalities

    Sinus bradycardia (HR < 50 bpm)

    Prolonged corrected Q-T interval

    Arrhythmias

- Physiologic instability

    Bradycardia

    Hypotension

    Hypothermia

> Orthostatic changes
>
> Syncope

- Arrested growth and development
- Failure of outpatient management (weight gain ½–1 pound/week)
- Intractable vomiting, binging or purging
- Acute food refusal
- Acute medical complication of malnutrition

  > Syncope
  >
  > Seizures
  >
  > Cardiac failure
  >
  > Pancreatitis

- Acute psychiatric emergency
  > Suicidal ideation
  >
  > Acute psychosis
- Comorbid diagnosis interfering with treatment
  > Severe depression
  >
  > Obsessive–compulsive disease (OCD)
  >
  > Severe family dysfunction
- Hospitalization
  > Can be medical or psychiatric ward
  >
  > Hospitalization until 90–92% of IBW
  >
  > For improved outcome need to gain 0.4 lb/day

Outpatient management

If none of the above characteristics present use outpatient therapy with multidisciplinary team:

Medical provider

> Coordinates care team
>
> Oversees treatment plan
>
> Manages medical issues:

- Weekly weigh in
- Vital sign stability
- Electrolyte/phosphorus abnormalities

- Hydration status
- Review objective physical findings with the patient, give clear information about growth, menses, osteopenia
- Acknowledge patient's distress: body image dissatisfaction vs nutritional needs
- Establish alliance with patient to work toward health
- Discuss reasons for hospitalization
- Review long-term goals

    Preventing osteopenia

    Preserving fertility

    Having a normal life

Dietitian with experience with anorexia

    Provide nutritional education

- Start with: 2–3 servings of protein/day; 30–50 g fat
- May increase fat slowly

    0–2 g/fat/week increase by 5 g per week to get to total of 30–50 g

Calcium: increase to 1200–1500 mg/day

Give specific caloric requirements: 1000–1600 kcal/day

Help plan appropriate weight goals: ½–2 pounds/week

Mental health professional

    Individual/cognitive behavioral therapy

    Family therapy

Pharmacotherapy

Anorexia

- Limited data with anorexia
- Consider treating comorbid disorders like depression or OCD
- In patients with anxiety, consider anxiolytic before meals
- Psychotropic medications not indicated as the sole or primary treatment for anorexia nervosa but fluoxetine can be considered for prevention of relapse in weight restored patients or to treat depression or OCD

Bulimia

- Drugs proven to decrease binge/purge activity:

    Fluoxetine 20–60 mg daily

Tricyclic antidepressants

Desipramine

Imipramine

Amitriptyline

Monoamine oxidase inhibitors

Buspirone

Complications

Watch for refeeding syndrome

- Definition:

    Congestive heart failure and resultant edema thought to be the result of hypophosphatemia associated with refeeding

- Management:

    Monitor phosphate levels, watch for signs of edema and congestive heart failure

    Patient at risk if < 10% IBW

    Consider phosphorus replacement while refeeding if patient with normal renal function

Watch for constipation/bloating

- Associated with refeeding
- May need metoclopramide and/or gastroenterology consult

Assess for osteopenia (see Osteoporosis, Chapter 38) for information on treatment with Actonel)

- One of the most severe complications of anorexia
- Estrogen replacement of limited success
- Treat with weight gain, 1200–1500 mg/day of calcium and 400 IU Vitamin D
- Dual emission X-ray absorptiometry (DEXA) at initial assessment and yearly

Long-term outcomes

50% – good outcome with return of menses and weight gain

25% – intermediate outcome: some weight gain and some relapse

25% – poor outcome: associated with later age onset of disorder, longer duration of illness and lower minimal weight

Mortality: 0.56% year (increases in mortality rate as duration of illness increases)

- Anorexics have a 10-fold increase in mortality vs unaffected
- Causes of death:

  54% – complications of anorexia

  27% – suicide

  19% – unknown or other causes

NATIONAL ORGANIZATIONS FOR EATING DISORDERS

American Anorexia Bulimia Association
165 W. 46th St.
Suite 1108
New York, NY 10036
212-575-6200
www.aabainc.org

National Association of Anorexia Nervosa and Associated Disorders
PO Box 7
Highland Park, IL 60035
847-831-3438
www.anad.org

Eating Disorders Awareness and Prevention
603 Steward Street Suite 803
Seattle, WA 98101
206-382-3587
800-931-2237
www.edap.org

BIBLIOGRAPHY

American Psychiatric Association. Practice guideline for the treatment of patients with eating disorders. *Am J Psychiatry* 2000;157(Suppl 1):1

Fisher M, Golden NH, Katzmann DK, *et al*. Eating disorders in adolescents: a background paper. *J Adolesc Health* 1995;16:420

Jimerson DC, Wolfe BE, Brotman AW, *et al*. Medications in the treatment of eating disorders. *Psychiatr Clin North Am* 1996;19:739

Kaye WH, Nagata T, Weltzin TE, *et al*. Double-blind placebo-controlled administration of fluoxetine in restricting and restricting-purging type anorexia nervosa. *Biol Psychiatry* 2000;49:644–52

Rome ES. Eating disorders in adolescents and young adults: what's a primary care clinician to do? *Cleveland Clin J Med* 1996;63:387

16 Emergency contraception (ECP)

KEY POINTS

Use of ECP decreases risk of pregnancy from 8% to 1–2% after a single episode of unprotected coitus

Most effective/tolerated agent is levonorgestrel (Plan B®)

An advance prescription ensures increased use of method over counseling alone

The closer to the sexual act the medication is taken the more effective

DIAGNOSIS

History

Unprotected coitus less than or equal to 120 hours previously?

Was last menstrual period normal? Was the previous menstrual period normal?

Current use of contraception and what method desired in the future

Physical examination/Laboratory tests

None required prior to ECP unless:

Suspicion of pregnancy: perform sensitive urine human chorionic gonadotropin (hCG) prior to treatment

Symptoms of sexually transmitted disease (STD): perform pelvic exam with STD screening

MANAGEMENT

Only hormonal methods appropriate for adolescents; avoid intrauterine device (IUD)

Pharmacologic methods

	#/color tablets to take within 120 h after unprotected coitus (the earlier more effective)	#/color tablets to take 12 h after the first dose
1. Plan B® (Women's Capitol Corp., Bellevue, WA) (0.75 mg levonorgestrel)	1 white	1 white
2.Yuzpe Preven® (Gynetics, Somerville, NJ) (levonorgestrel 0.25mg/ethinyl estradiol 50 µg)	2 blue	2 blue
Ovral® (Wyeth-Ayerst, Philadelphia, PA) (norgestrel 0.5 mg/ethinyl estradiol 50 µg)	2 white	2 white
Lo-Ovral® (Wyeth-Ayerst, Philadelphia, PA) (norgestrel 0.3 mg/ethinyl estradiol 30 µg)	4 white	4 white
Nordette® (Monarch, Bristol, TN) (levonorgestrel 0.15 mg/30 µg ethinyl estradiol)	4 light orange	4 light orange
Levlen® (Berlex, Wayne, NJ) (levonorgestrel 0.15mg/ethinyl estradiol 30 µg)	4 light orange	4 light orange
Levora® (Watson, Corona, CA) (levonorgestrel 0.15 mg/ethinyl estradiol 30 µg)	4 white	4 white
Triphasil® (Wyeth-Ayerst, Philadelphia, PA) (levonorgestrel 0.125 mg/ethinyl estradiol 30 µg)	4 yellow	4 yellow

Tri-Levlen® (Berlex, Wayne, NJ) (levonorgestrel 0.125 mg/ethinyl estradiol 30 µg)	4 yellow	4 yellow
Trivora® (Watson, Corona, CA) (levonorgestrel 0.125 mg/ethinyl estradiol 30 µg)	4 pink	4 pink
Alesse® (Wyeth-Ayerst, Philadelphia, PA) Levlite® (Berlex, Wayne, NJ) (levonorgestrel 0.1 mg/ethinyl estradiol 20 µg)	5 pink	5 pink
Ovrette® (Wyeth-Ayerst, Philadelphia, PA) (norgestrel 0.075 mg)	20 yellow	20 yellow

Contraindications

Consult before prescribing

For Plan B and Yuzpe: pregnancy, hypersensitivity to any component of product

For Yuzpe: history of/or current migraine with focal neurologic symptoms, previous thromboembolism

Side effects

	Yuzpe	Plan B®
Nausea	50%	23%
Vomiting	20%	6%
Bleeding	25%	25%
Fatigue	29%	17%
Dizziness	17%	11%
Breast tenderness	10–20%	11%

Other side effects for both methods include headache, abdominal pain/cramps

To manage the nausea: take with food; long acting emetics if taken one hour before the first dose, i.e. meclizine hydrochloride (OTC Dramamine, Pharmacia Consumer Healthcare, Peapack, NJ) or Bonine (Warner-Lambert, Morris Plains, NJ) one or two 25 mg tablets – may cause drowsiness

If vomiting occurs after a dose, replace the dose only if emesis occurs within one hour of a dose or if client can see the pills in the emesis

Menstrual bleeding may begin a few days earlier or a few days later than would have been expected

Effectiveness

Plan B® decreases the rate of pregnancy from 8% to 1% after a single act of coitus

Yuzpe decreases the rate of pregnancy from 8% to 2% after a single act of coitus

Either method is more effective the sooner it is utilized after a single act of coitus up to 120 hours

Follow-up

If menstrual bleeding does not occur within 3 weeks after treatment check for pregnancy

Ensure patient is using appropriate long-term contraception

HOW TO FIND AN ECP PROVIDER

Closest ECP provider: toll free 1-888-not-2-late

Closest Planned Parenthood Center: toll free 1-800-230-plan

Four states (Alaska, California, New Mexico, Washington) dispense EC without a prescription

Website dispenses for a fee: www.not-2-late.com

Plan B website: www.go2planb.com

Plan B telephone number: 800-330-1271

Preven website: www.preven.com

Preven telephone number: 888-Preven2 (888-773-8362)

BIBLIOGRAPHY

American College of Obstetricians and Gynecologists Practice Bulletin. *Emergency Oral Contraception*. Number 25, March 2001

17 EMLA® use, topical anesthetic

DEFINITION

Eutetic Mixture of Local Anesthetic agents (lidocaine 2.5% and prilocaine 2.5% in a 1 : 1 ratio with weight) for use as a topical anesthetic on normal intact skin

KEY POINTS

Useful as an adjunct for minor office dermatologic procedures in children (See Labial adhesions (Chapter 27) and Condyloma acuminatum (Chapter 10))

EMLA® CREAM INSTRUCTIONS

Apply EMLA® cream (AstraZeneca Pharmaceuticals LP, Wilmington, DE) and cover with an occlusive dressing (Tegaderm®, 3MHealthcare, St. Paul, MN) or another type, to achieve cutaneous anesthesia

After the allotted time (see below) wipe the cream off and proceed with procedure

Some specialists recommend instillation of 1% lidocaine subcutaneous after applying the EMLA® and before beginning the procedure to provide continued analgesia after the procedure is completed

Side effects/risks:

Local burning and erythema

Methemoglobinemia/lidocaine toxicity: slow speech, seizures, shallow respirations and other signs of central nervous system depression

Dosing:

Takes 30 min to 1 hour to achieve and may last up to 2 hours, providing topical anesthesia to a depth of 5 mm

Age dependent dose and maximal area of application:

Infant up to 3 months or < 5 kg:	1 g and 10 cm^2
Child 3–12 months and > 5 kg:	2 g and 20 cm^2
Child 1–6 years and > 10 kg:	10 g and 100 cm^2
Child 7–12 years and > 20 kg:	20 g and 200 cm^2

Maximum application time:

Infants < 3 months: one hour

Infants > 3 months: no longer than 4 hours

BIBLIOGRAPHY

Touma S, Jackson JB. Lidocaine and prilocaine toxicity in a patient receiving treatment for mollusca contagiosa. *J Am Acad Dermatol* 2001;44:399–400

18 Endometriosis

KEY POINTS

Adolescents typically present with pelvic pain

Most adolescents with endometriosis have both dysmenorrhea and pelvic pain

Endometriomas and infertility are rare presentations in the adolescent

Definitive diagnosis can only be established with laparoscopy with or without histologic confirmation of biopsy specimen

DEFINITION

Presence of endometrial glands and stroma outside the normal anatomic location of the lining of the uterus; located primarily in the pelvis in the adolescent (e.g. cul-de-sac, ovarian fossa)

PREVALENCE

Not clearly defined in available literature and may be underestimated

May be present in 67–73% of adolescents with chronic pelvic pain that is unresponsive to non-steroidal antiinflammatory drugs (NSAIDs) or oral contraceptive pills (OCPs)

Less commonly seen in 11–13 year olds than 20–21 year olds

May result from a polygenic/multifactorial inheritance pattern

PRESENTATION

Pelvic pain, dysmenorrhea in combination with acyclic pain

Cyclic pain, beginning 24–48 hours prior to menses, ends with cessation

Pain tends to increase in severity over time and may occur throughout the month

Initial relief of pain with NSAIDs/OCPs but then pain recurs

No correlation between extent of disease and severity of pain

Pain in patients with obstructive anomalies of the reproductive tract (e.g. imperforate hymen, vaginal septa)

Patients may have bowel or bladder symptoms

EVALUATION

(see Figure 18-1)

History

(See also Dysmenorrhea (Chapter 14) and Chronic pelvic pain (Chapter 44))

Review patient's pain

- Location, frequency, character of pain
- Relation to bowel/bladder function
- Cyclic or acyclic nature of pain
- Does the patient miss school/how much?
- Does the patient miss activities of daily living?
- Is pain worse with movement/better with rest?
- Endometriosis often associated with musculoskeletal pain

Family history

- Of endometriosis: 5-fold increased risk with 1st degree affected relative

Physical examination

(See also Chronic pelvic pain, Chapter 44)

Goal is to determine etiology for pain/rule out ovarian tumor/mullerian obstructive anomaly

In the non-sexually active teen, a recto-abdominal exam may be preferable

Occasionally rectal exam reveals cul-de-sac tenderness and rarely nodularity

Abdominal exam findings vary and can have a non-specific pattern of tenderness

Laboratory

Complete blood count (CBC), erythrocyte sedimentation rate (ESR):

- to rule out inflammatory process for pain

Urinalysis:

- to rule out urinary cause of pain

Sexually transmitted disease and pregnancy testing in the sexually active patient

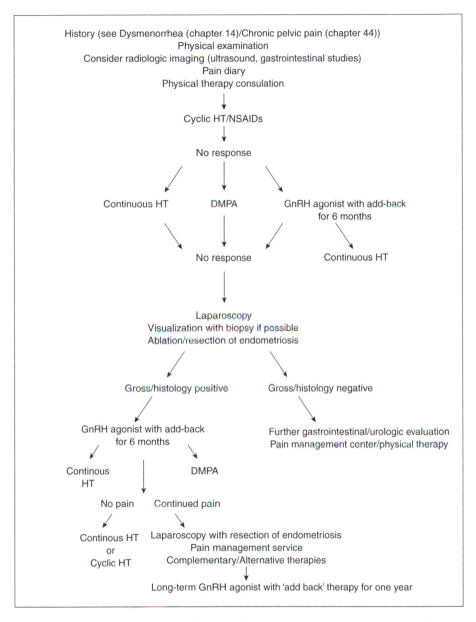

Figure 18-1   Management algorithm for the evaluation and treatment of pelvic/ pain endometriosis. HT, Hormonal therapy (oral contraceptive pill, estrogen/ progestin contraceptive patch, estrogen/progestin contraceptive ring, norethindrone acetate); NSAIDs, non-steroidal antiinflammatory drugs; DMPA, depot medroxyprogesterone acetate; GnRH, gonadotropin releasing hormone; Add-back, estrogen + progestin or norethindrone acetate alone Adapted with permission from Laufer MR, Sanfilippo JS, Rose G. Adolescent endometriosis: diagnosis and treatment approaches. *J Pediatr Adolesc Gynecol* 2003;16:S3–S11. © 2003 North American Society of Pediatric and Adolescent Gynecology

Imaging

Ultrasound

MRI if suspect mullerian anomaly

MANAGEMENT

Evaluate and treat for other etiologies of dysmenorrhea (e.g. hormonal therapy like OCPs and NSAIDs)

Consider endometriosis if pain still present

Surgery may eventually be necessary for definitive diagnosis but primary medical therapy has been advocated for presumed endometriosis in the adolescent

Either use empiric medical treatment with continuous OCPs/depot medroxyprogesterone acetate (DMPA) or gonadotropin releasing hormone (GnRH) agonist *or*

Make definitive diagnosis with surgery:

- Typically via laparoscopy
- Appearance may be atypical, clear or red vesicular lesions, white scarred areas, black implants or severe adhesive disease
- May help to visualize cul-de-sac through the laparoscope after filling with irrigation fluid to facilitate identification of vesicular lesions

The American Society for Reproductive Medicine is the accepted staging system standard to assist in comparing response to treatment (see Figure 18-2)

- Stage I: minimal disease, 1–5 points
- Stage II: mild disease, 6–15 points
- Stage III: moderate, 16–40 points
- Stage IV: severe, > 40 points

TREATMENT OPTIONS

Medical therapy

Use of hormonal therapy (HT) to create a hypoestrogenic environment which is not conducive to growth of endometriosis

Any of the following are acceptable:

AMERICAN SOCIETY FOR REPRODUCTIVE MEDICINE
REVISED CLASSIFICATION OF ENDOMETRIOSIS

Patient's Name _____   Date _____

Stage I   (Minimal)   – 1–5
Stage II   (Mild)   – 6–15   Laparoscopy _____ Laparotomy _____ Photography _____
Stage III (Moderate) – 16–40   Recommended Treatment _____
Stage IV (Severe)   – > 40   _____
Total _____   Prognosis_____

PERITONEUM	ENDOMETRIOSIS		< 1 cm	1–3 cm	> 3 cm
		Superficial	1	2	4
		Deep	2	4	6
OVARY	R	Superficial	1	2	4
		Deep	4	16	20
	L	Superficial	1	2	4
		Deep	4	16	20

	POSTERIOR CULDESAC OBLITERATION	Partial		Complete	
		4		40	

	ADHESIONS		< 1/3 Enclosure	1/3–2/3 Enclosure	> 2/3 Enclosure
OVARY	R	Filmy	1	2	4
		Dense	4	8	16
	L	Filmy	1	2	4
		Dense	4	8	16
TUBE	R	Filmy	1	2	4
		Dense	4*	8*	16
	L	Filmy	1	2	4
		Dense	4*	8*	16

*If the fimbriated end of the fallopian tube is completely enclosed, change the point assignment to 16.

Denote appearance of superficial implant types as red [(R), red, red-pink, flamelike, vesicular blobs, clear vesicles], white [(W), opacifications, peritoneal defects, yellow-brown], or black [(B) black, hemosiderin deposits, blue]. Denote percent of total described as R___%, W___% and B___%. Total should equal 100%

Additional Endometriosis: _____   Associated Pathology: _____
_____   _____

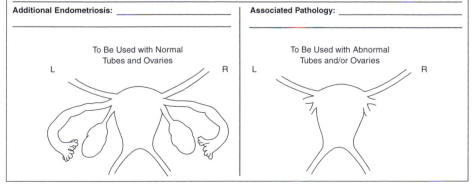

To Be Used with Normal   To Be Used with Abnormal
Tubes and Ovaries   Tubes and/or Ovaries
L   R   L   R

Figure 18-2   The American Society of Reproductive Medicine (formerly The American Fertility Society) Revised Classification of Endometriosis. © ASRM, 1997

EXAMPLES & GUIDELINES

STAGE I (MINIMAL)

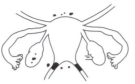

PERITONEUM
  Superficial Endo – 1–3 cm –2
R. OVARY
  Superficial Endo – < 1 cm –1
  Filmy Adhesions – < 1/3 –1
          TOTAL POINTS   4

STAGE II (MILD)

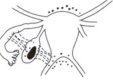

PERITONEUM
  Deep Endo   – > 3 cm –6
R. OVARY
  Superficial Endo – < 1 cm –1
  Filmy Adhesions – < 1/3 –1
L. OVARY
  Superficial Endo – < 1 cm –1
          TOTAL POINTS   9

STAGE III (MODERATE)

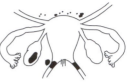

PERITONEUM
  Deep Endo   – > 3 cm –6
CULDESAC
  Partial Obliteration   –4
L. OVARY
  Deep Endo   – 1–3 cm –16
          TOTAL POINTS   26

STAGE III (MODERATE)

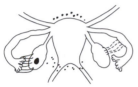

PERITONEUM
  Superficial Endo – > 3 cm –4
R. TUBE
  Filmy Adhesions – < 1/3 –1
R. OVARY
  Filmy Adhesions – < 1/3 –1
L. TUBE
  Dense Adhesions – < 1/3 –16*
L. OVARY
  Deep Endo   – < 1cm –4
  Dense Adhesions – < 1/3 –4
          TOTAL POINTS   30

STAGE IV (SEVERE)

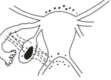

PERITONEUM
  Superficial Endo – > 3 cm –4
L. OVARY
  Deep Endo   – 1–3cm –32"
  Dense Adhesions – < 1/3 –8"
L. TUBE
  Dense Adhesions – < 1/3 –8"
          TOTAL POINTS   52

*Point assignment changed to 16
"Point assignment doubled

STAGE IV (SEVERE)

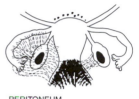

PERITONEUM
  Deep Endo   – > 3 cm   6
CULDESAC
  Complete Obliteration   –40
R. OVARY
  Deep Endo   – 1–3 cm –16
  Dense Adhesions – < 1/3   –4
L. TUBE
  Dense Adhesions – > 2/3   –16
L. OVARY
  Deep Endo   – 1–3 cm –16
  Dense Adhesions – > 2/3   –16
          TOTAL POINTS   114

Determination of the stage or degree of endometrial involvement is based on a weighted point system. Distribution of points has been arbitrarily determined and may require further revision or refinement as knowledge of the disease increases.

To ensure complete evaluation, inspection of the pelvis in a clockwise or counterclockwise fashion is encouraged. Number, size and location of endometrial implants, plaques, endometriomas and/or adhesions are noted. For example, five separate 0.5 cm superficial implants on the peritoneum (2.5 cm total) would be assigned 2 points. (The surface of the uterus should be considered peritoneum.) The severity of the endometriosis or adhesions should be assigned the highest score only for peritoneum, ovary, tube or culdesac. For example, a 4 cm superficial and a 2 cm deep implant of the peritoneum should be given a score of 6 (not 8). A 4 cm deep endometrioma of the ovary associated with more than 3 cm of superficial disease should be scored 20 (not 24).

In those patients with only one adenexa, points applied to disease of the remaining tube and ovary should be multipled by two. **Points assigned may be circled and totaled. Aggregation of points indicates stage of disease (minimal, mild, moderate, or severe).

The presence of endometriosis of the bowel, urinary tract, fallopian tube, vagina, cervix, skin etc., should be documented under "additional endometriosis." Other pathology such as tubal occlusion, leiomyomata, uterine, anomaly, etc., should be documented under "associated pathology." All pathology should be depicted as specifically as possible on the sketch of pelvic organs, and means of observation (laparoscopy or laparotomy) should be noted.

For additional supply wirte to: American Society for Reproductive Medicine,
1209 Montgomery Highway, Birmingham, Alabama 35216

American Society for Reproductive Medicine   *Revised ASRM classification: 1996*   *Fertility and Sterility®*

Oral contraceptive pills (OCPs)

Act to suppress the gonadotropic stimulation to the ovary and create a progestin dominant environment creating an atrophic endometrium

Can be used in the traditional 3-week fashion or as a continuous method to prevent menstrual flow. Take orally daily until patient experiences atrophic breakthrough bleeding or progestin side effects (bloating, weight gain, acne, headaches, emotional lability) occur. The timing of breakthrough bleeding and side effects will vary among individuals and will require cessation of OCPs for 7 days and restarting continuous therapy or alternatively, give for 2–3 months followed by a 4-day break for bleeding. Use a monophasic progestin-dominant pill such as Lo-Ovral (Wyeth-Ayerst, Philadelphia, PA)

Contraceptive patch (OrthoEvraâ, Ortho-McNeil Pharmaceutical Inc., Raritan, NJ) or vaginal ring (Nuvaringâ, Inc., West Orange, NJ)

Can be used cyclically or continuously as with OCPs

No current literature on use with endometriosis but threoretically would be similar to use of OCPs

Progestin

Commonly used regimens:

- Norethindrone acetate 15 mg by mouth daily
- Medroxyprogesterone acetate 30–50 mg by mouth daily
- Depot medroxyprogesterone acetate 150 mg intramuscularly every 1 to 3 months

Side effects are weight gain, bloating, acne, irregular bleeding

Used mainly in those who do not respond to OCPs or have contraindication to OCP use

Long term use of 1 or more years may be associated with decrease in bone mineral density and may require bone densitometry assessment

May be best utilized after a course of GnRH agonists

GnRH agonist

Use to induce a reversible hypoestrogenic state that removes the source of stimulation to the endometrial implants

Available as nasal spray, subcutaneous or intramuscular injection

Compliance is an issue in adolescents therefore intramuscular dosing more common

Typical dose: depot leuprolide (Lupron Depot, TAP Pharmaceuticals, Inc., Lake Forest, IL) 3.75 mg IM every 4 weeks

- Can also use 11.25 mg every 12 weeks

Usual therapy for 6 months then continue with OCPs or DMPA as above

Side effects:

- An induced agonist associated bleed 10–14 days after 1st use
- Osteopenia, hypoestrogenic symptoms like hot flashes, vaginal dryness
- Some patients may experience brownish menstrual spotting/ discharge due to shedding of atrophic endometrium

Add-back therapy: Use of estrogen and/or progestin to minimize GnRH agonist side effects and osteoporosis

- Progestin medication:

    Norethindrone acetate 5.0 mg po daily with start of GnRH agonist

    Has advantage of no stimulation of endometriosis with decrease in vasomotor symptoms and osteoporosis

- Estrogen and progestin:

    Norethindrone acetate 5.0 mg /day with conjugated equine estrogen 0.3 mg or 0.625 mg orally daily while on GnRH agonist

    Will decrease vasomotor symptoms, osteopenia, dyspareunia and vaginal atrophy but may stimulate endometriosis and/or retard its atrophy

Surgical therapy

Diagnostic and therapeutic laparoscopy:

- Gross resection, laser vaporization, endocoagulation or electrocoagulation of visible implants
- Goal is removal and destruction of all visible implants with lysis of adhesions, restoration of normal anatomy and preservation of reproductive organs
- There are no long-term studies on surgical outcomes in adolescents with endometriosis but resection studies in adults reveal 70–100% improvement of pain after surgical treatment
- While radical surgery of oophorectomy considered a possible treatment in adults, this is NOT indicated in the adolescent with endometriosis and pain

Chronic pain therapy

May need multidisciplinary approach for adolescents with endometriosis and chronic pelvic pain with referral to a pain center or clinic

- Analgesic/medication trials:

    Antidepressants: may have neuromodulatory/analgesic properties

    Amitriptyline 10–20 mg by mouth at bedtime

    Need baseline EKG before use to rule out preexisting prolonged QT or abnormal rhythm predisposing patients to rare sudden death with tricyclic antidepressant use

    Tramadol: centrally acting analgesic

    Cyclooxygenase-2 inhibitors:

    Celebrex (G.D. Searle & Co., Chicago, IL) and Vioxx (Merck, & Co., West Point, PA)

Cognitive–behavioral therapy:

- Assist patient with progressive muscle relaxation with pain

Physical therapy:

- To relieve associated myofascial pain
- Transcutaneous electric nerve stimulation (TENS)

Complementary/alternative therapies:

- Acupuncture

Websites: www.youngwomenshealth.org

www.endometriosisassn.org

BIBLIOGRAPHY

Greco C. Management of adolescent chronic pelvic pain from endometriosis: A pain center perspective. *J Pediatr Adolesc Gynecol* 2003;16:S17–S19

Hornstein MD, Surrey ES, Weisberg GW, *et al.* Leuprolide acetate depot and hormonal add-back in endometriosis: A 12-month study. Lupron Add-Back Study Group. *Obstet Gynecol* 1998;91:16–24

Laufer MR, Sanfilippo JS, Rose G. Adolescent endometriosis: diagnosis and treatment approaches. *J Pediatr Adolesc Gynecol* 2003;16:S3–S11

Propst AM, Laufer MR. Endometriosis in adolescents. Incidence, diagnosis and treatment. *J Reprod Med* 1999;44:751–8

19 Female circumcision

Collective name given to several different traditional practices that involve the cutting of female genitals

TYPES

(See Figure 19.1)

Type I or 'sunna' circumcision: removal of all or part of the clitoris; may cause sexual dysfunction but is associated with less long-term physical morbidity

Type II: excision of clitoris and a portion of labia minora, vagina uncovered

Type III or 'infibulation' or 'pharonic' circumcision: amputation of the clitoris, labia minora and medial portion of the labia majora, with subsequent suturing or chemical cauterization of the lateral aspects of wound in the midline; creates a flap or hood of smooth skin in front of the urethra and introitus; most immediate and long-term morbidity

PRESENTATION

Immediate: hemmorhage, severe pain, infection, lower urinary tract injuries, shock and death

Long-term: dysmenorrhea, dyspareunia, recurrent urinary or lower genital infections,voiding dysfunction; vulvar covering predisposes to vulvar irritation, infection, dribbling and vaginal calculus; significant keloid formation and/or sebaceous inclusion cysts along infibulated scar

Psychologic: anxiety, depression, sexual dysfunction

INTERVENTIONS

Reporting

The American College of Obstetricians and Gynecologists (ACOG) recommends that a Western provider who encounters a child who has

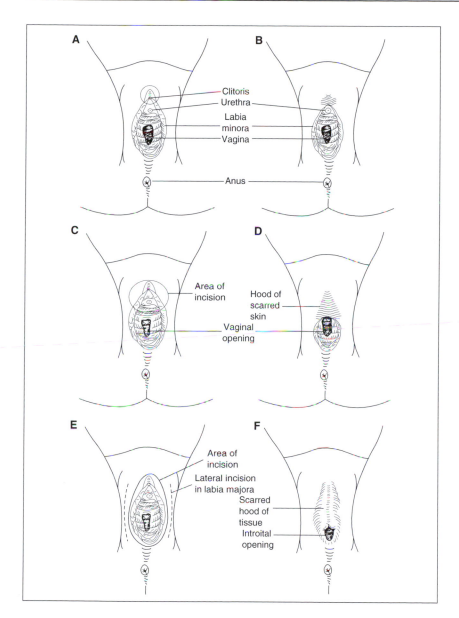

Figure 19-1 WHO Classification. **A, B:** Type I, removal of the clitoris. Part or whole of the clitoris is amputated. Stitching or pressure is used to control bleeding. **C, D:** Type II, excision. The clitoris and labia minora are amputated. Edges are sutured to control bleeding. The vagina is usually left exposed. **E, F:** Type III, infibulation. The clitoris and labia minora are removed. Incisions are made in the labia majora. The lateral raw surfaces are approximated, creating a hood of skin covering the urethra and vagina. Reproduced with permission from: The North American Society of Pediatric and Adolescent Gynecology. Strickland JL. Female circumcision/female genital mutilation. *J Pediatr Adolesc Gynecol* 2001;14:109–12. © 2001 North American Society of Pediatric and Adolescent Gynecology

recently been circumcised report to Child Protective Services as per their regional reporting standards

Counseling

It is important for the provider to recognize that this procedure is done in the context of caring and cultural norms and to relay that in counseling sessions

The provider should strongly discourage parents of children who are at risk from having the procedure, citing the morbidity as listed above

As adolescence is a time when feeling normal is of paramount importance, reassure the circumcised young woman that their appearance is normal for their native culture

Deinfibulation

Deinfibulation or incision of the covering of the hood of the tissue of Type III circumcised women should be considered before pregnancy, possibly before initiation of sexual activity

There is no Western legal precedent for the adolescent requesting confidential deinfibulation

Symptoms of dysmenorrhea, dyspareunia, recurrent urinary infections, and voiding dysfunction may be improved, even cured by deinfibulation

Deinfibulation procedure

To release the labia, either cold knife or CO_2 laser has been described

To prevent injury, it is helpful to place a moistened Q-tip inside the posterior vulvar opening and push it toward the top of the fusion line near the periclitoral area

Incision is made along the fusion line of the labia majora from the posterior vulvar opening to the periclitoral extreme

Careful hemostasis is essential; advantage of laser is that sutures are not required but this is very operator dependent

Suture material suggested is 4-0 or 5-0 Vicryl

Use of estrogen cream postoperatively may prevent scar and reformation

BIBLIOGRAPHY

Strickland JL. Female circumcision/female genital mutilation. *J Pediatr Adolesc Gynecol* 2001;14:109–12

20 Genital trauma

Maintain calm demeanor

Assess hemodynamic stability

Assess if history fits physical findings, i.e. type and extent of wound

Straddle injuries usually affect the labia and/or posterior fourchette

Penetrative injuries usually affect the vagina

Wounds that are attributable to sexual assault will often have other explanations

If sexual abuse is suspected or the injury does not fit the history, a report should be made to the appropriate law enforcement officials; if the injury occurred within 72 h of the visit a rape kit, forensic material collection and cultures/serologies for sexually transmitted diseases (STDs) should be obtained (see Sexual abuse, Chapter 54)

Assess ability to void

Assess for signs of intraabdominal injury

Assess need for repair of injury

MANAGEMENT

Repair of injury

Superficial genital lacerations and abrasions not actively bleeding:

- Coat with lidocaine jelly
- Rinse with warm water; helpful to use a large bore angiocath (14 French, 16 French) without the needle attached to a 20 ml syringe
- If still no active bleeding, observation
- Home care: sitz baths, warm water, tid to qid; minimal activity

Small vulvar hematomas which do not distort the anatomy or affect voiding:

- Ensure not expanding and no evidence of necrosis to surrounding tissue

- Home care: ice to area for 20–30 min qid for 48 h; then start sitz baths qid until resolves; minimal activity; supine position preferred

Bite wounds should be irrigated copiously and necrotic tissue cautiously debrided; non-infected fresh wound can often be closed primarily but most bite wounds should be left open with closure once granulation tissue formed

IF injury more than above, (i.e. less than hemostatic, deep, involves a hematoma that is affecting voiding or anatomy or overlying tissue is necrotic):

- Evaluate and treat under anesthesia. May need Foley catheter for assistance immediately postoperatively. Use absorbable sutures. Would not close a wound over 24 h old, would pack until hemostatic and/or begins to granulate in. Same homegoing instructions

If injury extends through or above the hymen, or was caused by a penetrating object whose length could extend into the peritoneal cavity:

- Perform CT or abdominal plain films to rule out intraabdominal and/or bony pelvis injury
- Complete comprehensive examination under anesthesia:

    Once anesthesia induced and prior to sterile prep, obtain forensic and STD specimens

    Make a careful anatomic description of the injury with photodocumentation if possible

    Perform vaginoscopy: see Operative care (Chapter 37)

    Perform cystoscopy and sigmoidoscopy by appropriate specialist if extensive injury warrants

    IF visualization is still compromised, small ribbon retractors with a headlight are helpful

    Ensure hemostasis; repair with fine absorbable suture material, i.e. 4-0 Vicryl

Additional therapy

Tetanus booster should be provided if none within five years

Broad-spectrum antibiotics should be used therapeutically not prophylactically

Postoperative visit

Repetitive reassurance that injuries will not affect the ability to have healthy sexual relations and bear children in the future should be brought up by the caregiver

Long-term morbidity rare even when there is an impalement injury with severe anogenital trauma

BIBLIOGRAPHY

Pokorny SF. Genital trauma. *Clin Obstet Gynecol* 1997;40:219–25

21 Gynecologic examination

PEDIATRIC PATIENT

NEWBORN/INFANT

Examination of the genitalia of a newborn should be routine in the delivery room

Location:	Isolette/exam table
Position:	Frog-leg position
Technique:	Labial separation/traction
	Perform gentle abdominal exam to palpate any masses
	(Pelvic masses i.e. ovarian cysts tend to be abdominal in infants due to their small bony pelvices)
Common findings:	
Newborn:	Maternal estrogenization (see Figure 21-1)
	Plump/full labia majora
	Mucous vaginal discharge
	Thick pale pink hymen
	Signs of estrogenization diminish after 2–3 weeks
Older infant:	Hypoestrogenic vulvar tissue (see Figure 21-1)
	Less prominent labia majora/minora
	Hymen recessed into vestibule appears thin/red

PREPUBERTAL FEMALE

Most gynecologic concerns at this age are:

- Concerns about anatomical development
- External epithelial conditions
- Vulvovaginitis

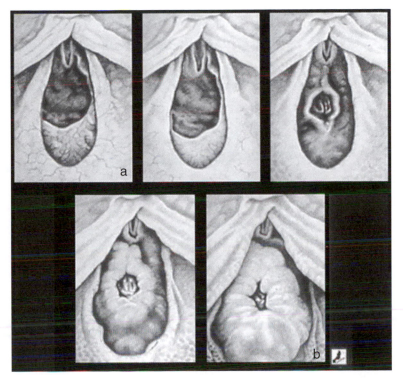

Figure 21-1 Progressive effects of estrogen on hymenal appearance: (a) Unestrogenized prepubertal appearance. (b) Estrogenized (neonatal/pubertal) appearance. Used with permission from the North American Society for Pediatric and Adolescent Gynecology. The PediGYN Teaching Slide Set. Elaine E Yordan, MD (ed)

History

Spend time during the history establishing a rapport with the young patient by including questions about family, best friends, favorite activities before performing exam

Explain the concept of the exam after obtaining history

Physical examination

Involve the patient in the exam to emphasize that they have some control

- Would you like to wear a blue gown or a green gown?
- Would you like to sit on your mom/dad's lap or on the table?

Perform a thorough exam

- Start by listening to heart and lungs while assessing body habitus/hygiene/skin disorders or discoloration and allow patient to feel comfortable

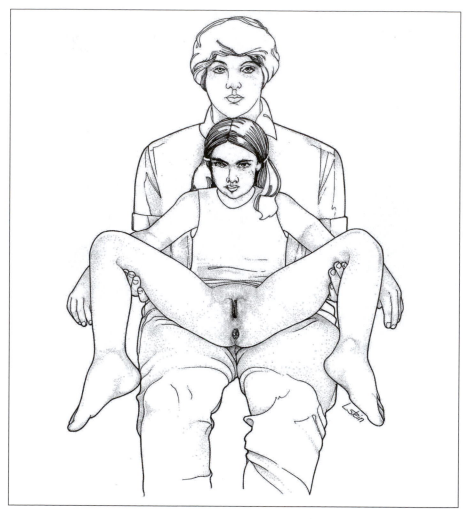

Figure 21-2 Child in supine frog-leg position while in mother's lap. Used with permission from Finkel MA, Giardino AP (eds). *Medical Evaluation of Child Sexual Abuse: A Practical Guide*, 2nd edn. Thousand Oaks, CA: Sage Publications, 2002;46–64. © Sage Publications, Inc.

Position the child appropriately for genitalia examination

- Most children over age 2 are able to use the stirrups or parent's lap for dorsolithotomy (see Figure 21-2)
- Frog leg (see Figure 21-3)
- Knee–chest position (see Figures 21-4, 21-5)

    Helpful adjunctive position

    May be able to visualize lower and even upper vagina with use of otoscope or ophthalmoscope

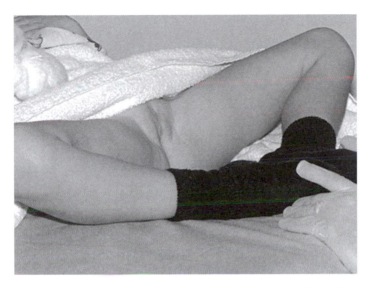

Figure 21-3 5-year-old demonstrating the supine 'frog-leg' position. Used with permission from McCann JJ, Kerns DL. *The Anatomy of Child and Adolescent Sexual Abuse*: A CD-ROM Atlas/Reference. St. Louis, MO: InterCorp, Inc.

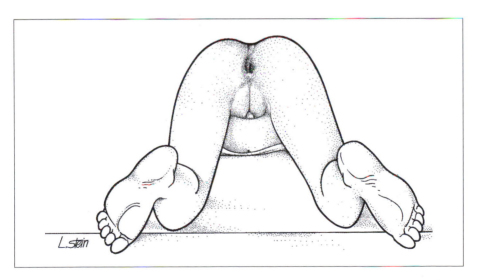

Figure 21-4 Child in prone knee–chest position for genital examination. Used with permission from Finkel MA, Giardino AP (eds). *Medical Evaluation of Child Sexual Abuse: A Practical Guide*, 2nd edn. Thousand Oaks, CA: Sage Publications, 2002;46–64. © Sage Publications, Inc.

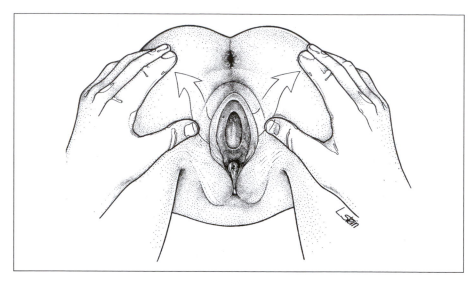

Figure 21-5 Technique for examination of female genitalia in prone knee–chest position. Used with permission from Finkel MA, Giardino AP (eds). *Medical Evaluation of Child Sexual Abuse: A Practical Guide*, 2nd edn. Thousand Oaks, CA: Sage Publications, 2002;46–64. © Sage Publications, Inc.

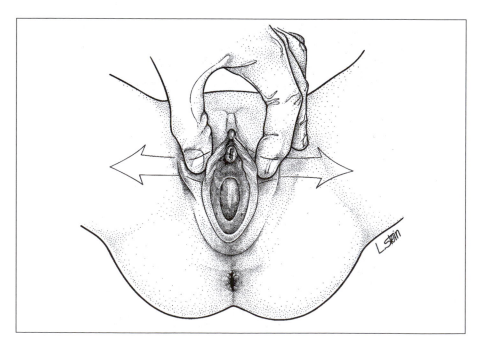

Figure 21-6 Labial separation technique for examination of femal genitalia in the supine frog-leg position. Used with permission from Finkel MA, Giardino AP (eds). *Medical Evaluation of Child Sexual Abuse: A Practical Guide*, 2nd edn. Thousand Oaks, CA: Sage Publications, 2002;46–64. © Sage Publications, Inc.

Visualize the vestibule:

- Labial separation (see Figure 21-6)
- Labial traction (see Figures 21-7, 21-8)

Assess:

- Presence of pubic hair (Tanner staging, see Figure 21-9)
- Clitoral size
- Hymenal shape (see figures showing hymenal shapes in Hymenal anatomy, Chapter 25)
- Signs of estrogenization (pale pink hymenal tissue vs reddened tissue)
- Presence or absence of vaginal discharge
- Perianal hygiene

Obtain specimens:

- Use small dacron swabs (male urethral size) to obtain vaginal swabs when necessary (see Figure 21-10)
- The prepubertal hymen is hypoestrogenic and sensitive to touch therefore consider using a 'catheter-within-a-catheter' technique by cutting a 4.5" butterfly catheter and putting it inside a #12 red rubber catheter attached to a 1-3 ml syringe to first instill 1 ml of fluid and then aspirate for use (Figure 21-11)

Document and describe findings:

- In prepubertal girls it is preferable to list each genital structure examined because future examiners will use the previous exams for the basis of their findings. This is particularly helpful in suspected abuse cases where a structure may have been altered by trauma, like a hymen
- List: labia majoral, labia minoral, hymenal shape or variations (bumps, clefts in hymen) urethral, vaginal, rectal findings even if normal (see Figure 21-12)
- It is helpful to use a clockface method to delineate location of any abnormal findings (see Figure 21-13)

Remember:

- Avoid iatrogenic trauma by not forcing exams on non-cooperative children
- Allow child to have sense of control by participating in exam (choosing gown, position for exam, putting on gloves)
- Tell the truth to children, if something will hurt, tell them it will hurt
- An examination under anesthesia may sometimes be necessary for patients who are non-compliant with exam

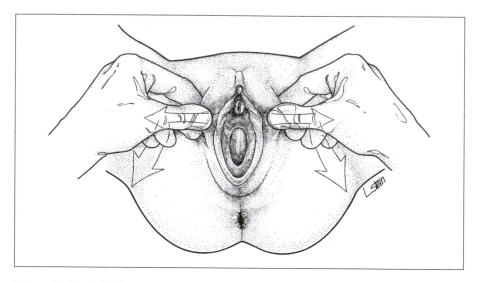

Figure 21-7 Labial traction technique for examination of female genitalia in the supine frog-leg position. Used with permission from Finkel MA, Giardino AP (eds). *Medical Evaluation of Child Sexual Abuse: A Practical Guide*, 2nd edn. Thousand Oaks, CA: Sage Publications, 2002;46–64. © Sage Publications, Inc.

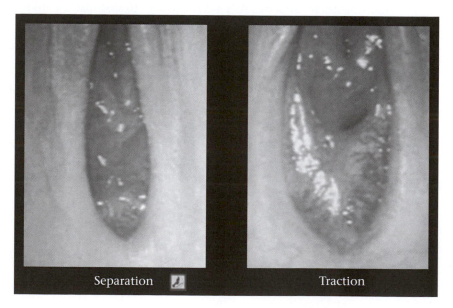

Figure 21-8 Examples of the techniques of labial separation and lateral traction for viewing the hymen of a prepubertal girl. Used with permission from the North American Society for Pediatric and Adolescent Gynecology. The PediGYN Teaching Slide Set. Elaine E Yordan, MD (ed)

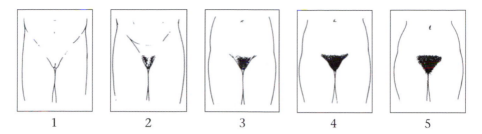

$$\begin{array}{ccccc} 1 & 2 & 3 & 4 & 5 \end{array}$$

Figure 21-9 Tanner stages: female pubic hair. Used with permission from Patient Care, May 30, 1979. © Medical Economics Co., Inc., Montvale, NJ. All rights reserved. Illustration by Paul Singh-Roy

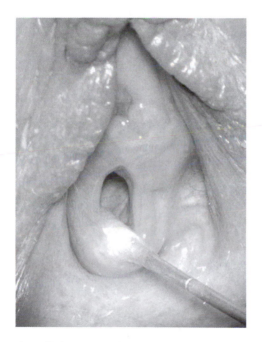

Figure 21-10 Use of small dacron swabs to obtain vaginal swabs. Used with permission from McCann JJ, Kerns DL. *The Anatomy of Child and Adolescent Sexual Abuse*: A CD-ROM Atlas/Reference. St. Louis, MO: InterCorp, Inc.

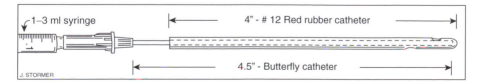

Figure 21-11 Assembled catheter-within-a-catheter, as used to obtain samples of vaginal secretions from prepubertal patients. Used with permission from Pokorny SF, Stormer J. A traumatic removal of secretions from the prepubertal vagina. *Am J Obstet Gynecol* 1987;156:581–2. © 1987 Mosby

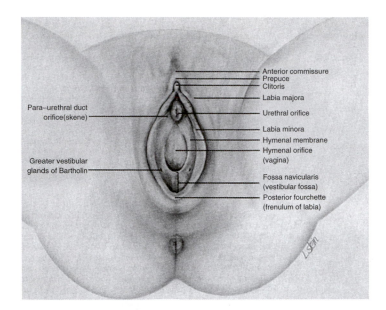

Figure 21-12 External structures of the female genitalia. Used with permission from Finkel MA, Giardino AP (eds). *Medical Evaluation of Child Sexual Abuse: A Practical Guide*, 2nd edn. Thousand Oaks, CA: Sage Publications, 2002;46–64. © Sage Publications, Inc.

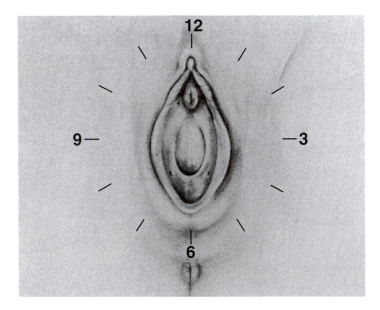

Figure 21-13 Face of clock orientation with patient in frog-leg supine position. Used with permission from Finkel MA, Giardino AP (eds). *Medical Evaluation of Child Sexual Abuse: A Practical Guide*, 2nd edn. Thousand Oaks, CA: Sage Publications, 2002;46–64. © Sage Publications, Inc.

ADOLESCENT PATIENT

INDICATIONS FOR ADOLESCENT GYN EXAM

Preventative visits:

- Age 13–15: Initial visit; does not necessarily include pelvic exam
- Yearly visits thereafter; pelvic when indicated

Annual/semi-annual for sexually active teens:

- Need sexually transmitted disease (STD) screening with each new partner
- Annual if regular partner

Indications for pelvic examination:

- Pubertal aberrancy
- Abnormal bleeding
- Abdominal or pelvic pain

Adolescents want confidentiality from their clinicians and for the clinician to ask the questions they won't (about STDs, contraception, acne, weight, menses, how their bodies work, and sexual behaviors like kissing, petting, intercourse)

Consider use of the American College of Obstetricians and Gynecologists (ACOG) Tool Kit for Teen Care that contains a confidential screening questionnaire to be used with each visit and an adolescent specific history and physical exam record (www.acog.org). (See Figure 21-14)

HISTORY HINTS

Start history by building trust with a friendly, respectful greeting:

'How may I help you today?'

Avoid 'What's your problem today?'

Meet initially with teen and her parents if possible

Explain concept of confidentiality and privacy to both parents and teen (ACOG has a helpful document on this topic in the Tool Kit (Figure 21-14))

Take sensitive part of history from teen without presence of parent (alcohol, drug and substance use, dating and sexual history)

When asking questions of teens:

Give a range of acceptable answers:

- 'Some teens can talk about sex with their parents; others can't. How do you feel?'

Create a context for questions:

- 'A lot of girls your age ... how do you feel about that?'

When screening, begin with less sensitive issues:

- Safety and education before affect and sexuality

Routine history: chief complaint, history of present illness, past medical history, family and social history

Gynecologic history:

Menarche – Average age of 1st period is 12.8 years

- Typically occurs about 2 years after breast budding occurred

Flow length – Usually 5–7 days, more than 10 requires evaluation

Interval between menses – Usually 21–35 days apart

First 1–2 years after menarche, cycles may be irregular

It may be 2–3 years before ovulation is routine and menses are regular

Heavy flow at menarche resulting in anemia is a sign of a bleeding disorder:

- Consider workup for von Willebrand's disease, platelet dysfunction

Any associated menstrual symptoms:

- Pain unrelieved with NSAIDs; nausea, vomiting, diarrhea
- Missed school due to menstrual symptoms
- Ask about family history of endometriosis if significant history of dysmenorrhea

    There is a 5-fold increase in endometriosis if 1st degree relative with endometriosis

Sexual history:

- Ask about age at first intercourse and whether consensual or forced
- Ask about number of partners, current partner
- Ask about method of birth control and use of condoms for STD protection

EXAMINATION

Pelvic examination

Explain process of exam before performing

Position:

- Use semi-sitting dorsolithotomy (lift back of exam table to allow better eye contact with provider giving better sense of control)
- Consider using mirror to show genital anatomy to patient

Inspect:

- External genitalia (Tanner staging)
- Vaginal/cervical exam (when indicated)

    Use appropriate size speculum

    Virginal/nulliparous patients – Huffman specula (1/2 × 4 inches long) (see Figure 21-15)

    Sexually active teens – Huffman or Pederson specula (7/8 × 4 inches long)

- Pap test (see Pap Testing)

    Within 3 years of onset of sexual activity

    Consider at presentation IF:

    Multiple partners

    HIV positive/immunocompromized status

    Patient not likely to comply with follow-up visits

- STD testing (see Sexually transmitted diseases, Chapter 56)

    Endocervical testing for chlamydia and gonorrhea, if sexually active

    If no pelvic exam completed, may do urine screening for chlamydia/gonorrhea

Bimanual exam (when indicated)

- Put single finger in the vagina/may use two fingers if patient parous
- Palpate cervix evaluating for cervical motion tenderness
- Assess uterine size and position (ante or retroverted)
- Assess adnexa for tenderness, masses, ovarian enlargement

- Perform rectovaginal bimanual exam

    For patients with abdominal pain or severe dysmenorrhea

    Assess cul-de-sac area for nodularity indicating endometriosis

    Assess for adnexal masses, uterine anomalies

    Consider hemoccult testing of stool in patients with abdominal pain

Hints on conveying information

After the exam:

- **In the non-sexually active teen** – meet with family member and patient together to review findings and make plan

- **In the sexually active teen, if confidentiality is a concern** – first discuss findings with patient alone while in the examination room. Make a plan together about how to discuss with parent/guardian. Encourage the teen to allow you to be the liaison between her and her family stressing the benefits of informing everyone of contraception use and her situation. Then meet together with family.

After discussions about outcome of the exam and findings, when it is time to make a decision between medical therapies – make it clear that a decision is needed and that the decision belongs to the patient not to the parent

Ask: 'What have you decided to do?'

If any indecision, indicates need for further discussion

Reflecting patient's decision back can often clarify situation:

- 'So, you have decided to …' then allow patient to agree or disagree

When providing instructions:

- Give, short, simple, repetitive instructions

- Make links for taking medicine 'When brush teeth, take pill'

- Check understanding by having teen repeat back to you

- Send printed instructions home

Encourage follow up by anchoring experience to external events:

- 'Come back during week of Thanksgiving' instead of 'end of November'

ADOLESCENT VISIT QUESTIONNAIRE

We strongly encourage you to discuss all issues of your life with your parent(s) or guardian(s). However, unless it is a life threatening issue, the information you give us on this form is confidential between our doctors and nurses and you. It will not be released without your written consent. If you would like help filling out this form, please let the nurse know. IF YOU DON'T FEEL COMFORTABLE ANSWERING A QUESTION, LEAVE IT BLANK AND YOUR DOCTOR OR NURSE WILL TALK WITH YOU ABOUT IT.

Name _____   Age _____   Today's Date _____

Why did you come into our office today? _____

Please answer these general health questions. Ignore the last column. Your doctor or nurse will fill that out.

		For doctor/nurse use
Friends and Family		
Can you talk with your parent(s) or guardian(s) about personal things happening in your life?	❏ Yes ❏ No	
If no, is there another adult you trust and can talk to if you have a problem?	❏ Yes ❏ No Who?	
Who do you live with? (Please circle all that apply.)	Mother Father Guardian Sibling(s) Other:	
Do you think your family has lots of fun together?	❏ Yes ❏ No	
Do you think your parents care about you?	❏ Yes ❏ No	
Do you have a best friend?	❏ Yes ❏ No	
School and Work		
Do you like school and do well in school?	❏ Yes ❏ No ❏ Not in school	
What grade are you in?	Grade: ❏ Not in school	
What school do you go to?	School: ❏ Not in school	
How often have you skipped school?	❏ Never ❏ Once or twice ❏ A lot	
Do you have any learning problems?	❏ Yes ❏ No	
Do you have a job?	❏ Yes ❏ No Doing what?	
Do you know what you want to be when you are older?	❏ Yes ❏ No What?	
Appearance and Fitness		
Do you have any concerns or questions about the shape or size of your body or the way you look?	❏ Yes ❏ No ❏ Not sure	
Do you want to gain or lose weight?	❏ Gain ❏ Lose ❏ Neither	
Have you ever tried to lose weight or control your weight by throwing up, using diet pills or laxatives, or not eating for a day?	❏ Yes ❏ No	
Have you ever had your body pierced (other than ears) or gotten a tattoo?	❏ Yes ❏ No ❏ Considering	
Do you exercise or do a sport at least 5 times a week that makes you sweat or breathe hard for 30 minutes?	❏ Yes ❏ No	
How many fruits and vegetables do you eat each day?	❏ None ❏ 1–2 ❏ 3–4 ❏ 5–6 ❏ 7 or more	
How much milk, yogurt, ice cream do you eat each day?	❏ None ❏ 1–2 ❏ 3–4 ❏ 5–6 ❏ 7 or more	
Safety/Weapons/Violence		
Do you wear a seat belt when you ride in a car, truck, or van?	❏ Yes ❏ No	
Do you wear a helmet when you use a bike, motorcycle, all-terrain vehicle, mini-bike, skateboard, rollerblades, or scooter?	❏ Yes ❏ No	
Do you or does anyone you live with have a gun, rifle, or other firearm?	❏ Yes ❏ No ❏ Not sure	
Have you ever carried a gun or weapon?	❏ Yes ❏ No	
Have you ever been in trouble with the law?	❏ Yes ❏ No	
Has anyone touched you in a way that made you uncomfortable?	❏ Yes ❏ No ❏ Not sure	
Has anyone ever forced you to have sex?	❏ Yes ❏ No ❏ Not sure	
Has anyone ever hurt you physically or emotionally?	❏ Yes ❏ No ❏ Not sure	

Figure 21-14   ACOG Adolescent Visit Record and ACOG Adolescent Visit Questionnaire. Reproduced with permission from American College of Obstetricians and Gynecologists. *Tool Kit for Teen Care*. Washington, DC. © ACOG, 2003. Copies may be purchased at www.sales.acog.org

ADOLESCENT VISIT QUESTIONNAIRE *(continued)*

Relationships		For doctor/nurse use
Are you going out with anyone?	❏ Yes ❏ No	
Who do you find yourself attracted to sexually?	❏ Guys ❏ Girls ❏ Both	
Have you ever had sex with anyone? If yes, answer the questions in this section below.	❏ Yes ❏ No	
If no, do you plan to in the next year? When done answering this question, go to the section on tobacco, alcohol, and drugs below.	❏ Yes ❏ No ❏ Not sure	
How many sexual partners do you have now? How many in the past?	Now: Past:	
How old were you the first time you had sex (intercourse)?	Age:	
Have you ever had sex with a person of your same sex?	❏ Yes ❏ No	
Do you use anything to prevent pregnancy?	❏ Yes ❏ No If yes, what do you use?	
Do you and your partner(s) always use a condom when you have sex?	❏ Yes ❏ No	
Do you ever have sex for money or drugs?	❏ Yes ❏ No	
Are you worried about your parents knowing that you are having sex?	❏ Yes ❏ No	
Do you ever participate in other sexual activities, such as touching or oral or anal sex?	❏ Yes ❏ No	
If yes, do you use anything to prevent disease?	❏ Yes ❏ No If yes, what do you use?	
Tobacco, Alcohol, and Drugs		
Have you or your close friends ever smoked cigarettes or cigars, used snuff, or chewed tobacco?	❏ Yes, I have ❏ No, I haven't ❏ Yes, friends have ❏ No, friends haven't	
Have you or your close friends ever gotten drunk on wine, beer, or alcohol?	❏ Yes, I have ❏ No, I haven't ❏ Yes, friends have ❏ No, friends haven't	
How much alcohol do you drink at one time?	❏ Don't drink ❏ 1–2 glasses ❏ 3 or more	
Do you ever drink more than 5 drinks in a row?	❏ Don't drink ❏ Yes ❏ No	
In the last year, have you been in a car or other motor vehicle when the driver is drunk or has been drinking alcohol or using drugs? (This includes when you were the driver as well as other people.)	❏ Yes ❏ No	
Would you call your parent(s) or guardian(s) for a ride if you were stranded because the person who was supposed to drive you home had been drinking? (This includes when you were the driver as well as other people.)	❏ Yes ❏ No ❏ Not sure	
Have you or your close friends ever used marijuana or other drugs (like cocaine, heroin, or ecstasy) or sniffed inhalants?	❏ Yes, I have ❏ No, I haven't ❏ Yes, friends have ❏ No, friends haven't ❏ Not sure	
Have you ever used alcohol or drugs so much that you could not remember what happened?	❏ Don't use drugs or alcohol ❏ Yes ❏ No	
Have you ever missed work or school because of use of alcohol or drugs?	❏ Don't use drugs or alcohol ❏ Yes ❏ No	
Emotions		
In the past few weeks, have you often felt sad and down or as though you have nothing to look forward to?	❏ Yes ❏ No	
Have you ever seriously thought about killing yourself, made a plan or actually tried to kill yourself?	❏ Yes ❏ No	
During the past year, have you had any major good or bad changes in your life (death of someone close, birth, graduation, significant change in close relationship)?	❏ Good ❏ Bad ❏ No changes	

What would you like to discuss with our nurses and doctors today?_____

_____

Select questions have been taken directly or adapted from the following sources with permission. GAPS. Younger Adolescent Questionnaire. American Medical Association 1998. Available at http://www.ama-assn.org/ama/pub/category/2280.html. Retrieved May 8, 2002. Middle-Older Adolescent Questionnaire. American Medical Association 1997. Available at http://www.ama-assn.org/ama/pub/category/2280.html. Retrieved May 8, 2002.

Date: _____ Name: _____   Patient Addressograph
                                  LAST   FIRST   MIDDLE

Date of Birth:_____ Record Number:_____

Primary Physician: _____ Referral Source: _____

Insurance Carrier/Medicaid No.: _____

ACOG ADOLESCENT VISIT RECORD

I. General Information

Current age: Current medications:	Complaint(s), if any:

Contact information
(It should be determined who is aware of the teens sexual activity as this may affect where and/or how the teen wishes to be contacted with abnormal findings.)

II. History

FOR PROBLEM VISIT ONLY—History of Present Illness (HPI) (please describe, if any):	FOR PROBLEM VISIT ONLY—HPI elements: ☐ Location ☐ Severity ☐ Timing ☐ Modifying factors ☐ Quality ☐ Duration ☐ Context ☐ Associated signs and symptoms

Menstrual History

	Response	Details/Notes		Response	Details/Notes
Age at menarche			Last menstrual period		
Length of periods			Normal/Abnormal		
Cycle length			Cramping		

Past Medical and Family History

Past Medical History	(+) Pos (0) Neg	Details/Remarks
Past illnesses (measles, mumps, rheumatic fever, chicken pox, hepatitis, cancer, sickle cell anemia)		
Pulmonary (pneumonia, TB/lived with someone who has/had TB, asthma)		
Surgical procedures		
Trauma/violence		
Injuries/accidents		
Hospitalization		
Allergies		
Blood transfusions		
Previous cervical cytology Date:		Normal/Abnormal/ _____
Past family history		
Blood clots		
Parent with cholesterol >240		
Parent/grandparent death from heart attack/stroke at <55 years, coronary artery disease, peripheral vascular disease, cerebrovascular disease		
Ethnic background related diseases (Tay–Sachs, sickle cell anemia, Thalessemia)		
Cancer		
Diabetes		

A nurse or nursing assistant, depending on staff capabilities and facilities, can complete all shaded areas of the record.

Past Social History	Details/Notes
If sexually active, contraception/STD prevention method: Frequency of method use: _____ Number of current partners: _____ Age of initial coitus: _____ Number of past partners:_____ Pregnancies: G _____ P _____ AB _____ STDs, including herpes simplex virus: _____	SAMPLE

CPT Levels of History

Levels of History	Chief Complaint (CC)	History of Present Illness (HPI)	Review of Systems (ROS)	Past, Family, Social History (PFSH)
Problem focused	Required	Brief	Not required	Not required
Expanded problem focused	Required	Brief	Problem pertinent	Not required
Detailed	Required	Extended	Extended	Pertinent
Comprehensive	Required	Extended	Complete	Complete

III. Immunization

Routine (a check mark indicates a positive response)	Notations
☐ Tetanus Diphtheria (ideal booster at age 11–12, if not previously vaccinated within 5 years)	
☐ Measles-mumps-rubella (ideal second dose at age 11–12, unless 2 vaccinations in early childhood)	
☐ Hepatitis B vaccination (to be given at age 11–12, if previous recommended doses were missed)	
As indicated	
☐ Hepatitis A (traveling/living in endemic community, chronic liver disease, or injecting drug users)	
☐ Varicella vaccination (administered at age 11–12 to all unvaccinated patients or those lacking reliable history of chicken pox (susceptible patients age ≥ 13 receive 2 doses, at least 1 month apart)	

IV. Health Guidance/Counseling

Positive from Adolescent Visit Questionnaire:	Details/Notes	Positive from Adolescent Visit Questionnaire:	Details/Notes
Routine as appropriate		Routine as appropriate	
Tobacco		Emergency contraception	
Alcohol and other drugs		STDs, including HIV/AIDS	
Drinking and driving[1]		Sexual victimization risk reduction[2]	
Diet (calcium, weight management, folic acid)		Pregnancy counseling (options, prenatal care, school)	
Exercise		Violence	
Responsible sexual behavior (abstinence/contraception)		Conflict resolution	
Condoms (how to acquire, use, and talk with partner)		Seat belts/helmets	
Other		Other	

[1] Encourage adolescents and their parents to develop agreements for picking up adolescents who have consumed alcohol or other substances.
[2] Discuss role of alcohol and other drugs.

V. Vital Signs

Weight	Height	Blood Pressure
BMI[3]	Temperature	Pulse

[3] Body mass index is computed as weight (in kilograms) divided by height in meters squared. Using pounds and inches, multiply the division results by 700. To determine prepregnancy weight-for-height status, go to the BMI chart.

A nurse or nursing assistant, depending on staff capabilities and facilities, can complete all shaded areas of the record.

VI. Review of Systems

Systems	(+) Pos (0) Neg	Details/Notes
Constitutional (weight loss/gain, eating disorder)		
Eyes		
Ears, nose, mouth or throat problems		
Cardiovascular		
Respiratory		
Gastrointestinal (eating behaviors indicating an eating disorder)		
Genitourinary (urination problems, vaginal discharge)		
Musculoskeletal (muscle/joint pain, scoliosis, broken bones)		
Integumentary (severe acne)		
Breast tenderness, mass		
Neurologic (seizures/epilepsy, headaches/migraines)		
Psychiatric disorders (depression)		
Endocrine		
Hematologic/lymphatic (blood disorder, anemia)		
Allergic/immunologic		

VII. Physical Examination. Leave blank if not examined (required if history indicates and at least once at ages 12–14, 15–17, and 18–21)

Body Area/Organ System	Normal	Abnormal	Details/Notes	Body Area/Organ System	Normal	Abnormal	Details/Notes
Abdomen (masses, tenderness, hernia, HSM)				Genitourinary			
Extremities				Breasts Tanner stage:			
Neck (thyroid, masses)				Pubic Hair Tanner stage:			
Cardiovascular (peripheral system/auscultation)				Vulva/external genitalia			
Ears/Nose/Mouth/Throat (teeth)				Kidney/bladder			
Eyes				Vagina			
Gastrointestinal (digital rectal exam)				Uterus			
Hematologic/Lymphatic/ Immunologic (lymph nodes)				Adnexa			
Musculoskeletal				Anus/perineum			
Neurologic				Cervix			
Psychiatric				Urethral Meatus			
Respiratory (effort, auscultation)				Urethra			
Skin							

CPT Levels of Physical Examination

Level of Physical Examination	CPT Definitions
Problem focused	Limited examination of affected body area or organ system
Expanded problem focused	Limited examination of affected body area or organ system AND other symptomatic or related organ systems
Detailed	Extended examination of affected body area(s) AND other symptomatic or related organ systems
Comprehensive	General multi-system examination OR complete examination of single organ system

A nurse or nursing assistant, depending on staff capabilities and facilities, can complete all shaded areas of the record.

VIII. Testing Ordered/Performed

	Tests	Date	Results
General	Cholesterol[1] Lipoprotein profile[2] Tuberculin[3]		
Gynecologic	Cervical cytology[4] Gonorrhea[5] Chlamydia[6] Syphilis[6] HIV[7]		
Other			

[1]Adolescents with parental cholesterol >240 mg/dL should be screened for total blood cholesterol (nonfasting) at least once. Adolescents with either unknown family history, or multiple risk factors may be screened for total serum cholesterol level (nonfasting) at least once.
[2]Adolescents with parent/grandparent with coronary artery disease, peripheral vascular disease, cerebrovascular disease, or sudden cardiac death age <55 should be screened with a fasting lipoprotein profile.
[3]If have been exposed to active tuberculosis; have lived in a homeless shelter, been incarcerated, or lived in another long-term care facility; have lived in endemic area; currently working in health care setting; HIV positive; medically underserved or low-income; have history of alcoholism; have medical risk factors known to increase risk of disease if infected.
[4]Cervical cytology should be obtained no later than 3 years after first intercourse.
[5]Routine screening for chlamydial and gonorrheal infection should be performed for all sexually active adolescents.
[6]Serologic testing for syphilis should be conducted on sexually active adolescents who have a history of prior STDs, multiple sexual partners, exchanged sex for drugs or money, used illicit drugs, been admitted to jail or other detention facility, lived in an endemic area.
[7]Adolescents with the following risk factors should be offered HIV testing: multiple sexual partners, high-risk partner, prior STDs, exhanges sex for drugs or money, long-term residence or birth in an area with high prevalence of HIV infection, history of blood transfusion prior to 1985, use of intravenous drugs.

IX. Assessment/Plan

Assessment	Plan

FOR PROBLEM VISIT ONLY—CPT Level of Medical Decision Making (Two of the three required elements must be met or exceeded.)

Elements Included in Medical Decision Making Component			
Number of diagnoses or management options	Amount and/or complexity of data to be reviewed	Risk of complications and/or morbidity or mortality	Type of medical decision making
Minimal	Minimal or none	Minimal	Straightforward
Limited	Limited	Low	Low complexity
Multiple	Moderate	Moderate	Moderate complexity
Extensive	Extensive	High	High complexity

FOR PROBLEM VISIT ONLY—If E/M Code selected based on time:

Time spent counseling:	Physician signature:
Total time with patient:	

Box 1. Confidential Agreement

Parent

I, _____ (parent or guardian), allow

_____ (patient), to enter a confidential patient–physician relation-
ship. I understand that she can make independent health care decisions, but that my input and involvement will be encouraged.

_____ (patient)has permission to schedule appointments and
receive confidential reports from this office. I further understand that various laboratory tests may be
necessary in medical protocols and accept responsibility for physician charges and laboratory fees.

_____

Parent or Guardian

_____

Physician

Patient

I, _____ (patient), am entering a confidential physician–patient
relationship with

_____ (physician). I will make an effort to communicate with my
parent(s) or guardian(s) about issues concerning my health. I accept the personal responsibility of being
honest and will follow the health care recommendations my physician and I establish.

_____

Patient

_____

Physician

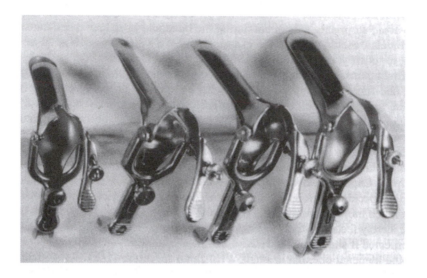

Figure 21-15   Types of specula (from left to right): infant, Huffman, Pederson, and Graves. Used with permission from Emans SJ. Office evaluation of the child and adolescent. In Emans SJ, Laufer MR, Goldstein DP (eds). *Pediatric and Adolescent Gynecology*, 4th edn. Philadelphia: Lippincott-Raven Publishers, 1998

22 Hemangioma of vulva

Unusual but well-recognized, more common in females

Majority will undergo spontaneous involution by age 5

Important to discern from vascular malformation:

> Hemangiomas are benign tumors of infancy and childhood – infancy with rapid growth of endothelial cells; childhood with slow spontaneous involution

> Vascular malformations comprise dysplastic vessels and never regress

DIAGNOSIS

Presentation may range from a small almost negligible vascular papule to massive distorting tumors

If diagnosis unclear, consider radiologic evaluation and/or consultation with a pediatric (or dermatologic, plastic, vascular) surgeon

> Ultrasound with color Doppler imaging is helpful, but extremely operator dependent due to the level of experience with this pediatric anomaly

> MRI is very useful but it usually requires sedation; it is best when the hemangioma has grown through the various tissue layers under the skin

> **Do not biopsy**

MANAGEMENT

Despite the size the majority will regress with time and either disappear or leave a small, mainly fibrosed tumor which may be removed at a safer age if necessary

Parents need to be cautioned to wait rather than have the child treated; this may be difficult for the child and parents, who may need significant support and consultations during this process. Pictures are helpful to follow the progression of involution

May be helpful to show examples of regression of hemangiomas in similar locations

Indications for treating hemangiomas during their growth phase:

Major expansion with disfigurement

Functional compromise, necrosis and ulceration

Options for treating hemangiomas during their growth phase (in order of increasing morbidity):

Oral corticosterioid (Prednisone 2–3 mg/kg/day) with full dosages in morning usually over a period of 6 weeks then slowly tapering over two months; good involution response rate in 30%

Interferon alpha used after failure of corticosteroids; good involution rate 75–80% of cases

Therapeutic embolization uses after medical treatment failure

Early surgical excision: will probably leave a scar which should be acceptable

Laser can be used to accelerate lightening and involution of superficial hemangiomas

BIBLIOGRAPHY

Enjolras O. Management of hemangiomas. *Dermatol Nurs* 1997;9:11–17

23 High risk behaviors

KEY POINTS

Appropriate preventative care for the adolescent includes annual assessment of both risk factors and protective factors in adolescent's life including the adolescent's attitude about substance use, teenage sexual practices, and education about negative consequences from high risk behaviors

DIAGNOSIS

Meet with parent and patient initially to identify reason for the visit then excuse the parent for the duration of the interview

As with any adolescent encounter, confidentiality should be defined, discussed and guaranteed as far as the practitioner is able with both the parent and child (See Confidentiality agreement, page 117). In all 50 states there is a guarantee of adolescent rights to seek help and intervention for substance abuse without parental involvement. If the clinician feels the adolescent is at high risk of harm that confidentiality should be relinquished.

Confidential interview: relaxed; listening actively; avoiding being judgmental responses; being straightforward and respectful

Screening tool can be filled out by the adolescent (see Figure 21-14: the self-administered confidential adolescent visit questionnaire) or by the practitioner (**HEADSFIRST** Screening Tool):

- H: Home – relationships, space, freedom and restrictions, support
- E: Education/employment – expectations, study habits, future, achievement, jobs
- A: Abuse – physical, sexual, emotional, verbal neglect
- D: Drugs – tobacco, alcohol, illicit drugs
- S: Safety – hazardous activities, seatbelts, helmets, driving
- F: Friends – confidant, peer pressure, interaction
- I: Image – self-esteem, appearance, body image, nutrition
- R: Recreation – exercise, relaxation and sleep, media use, sports

S: Sexuality – sexual identity, feelings, relationships, activity, safety, body changes

T: Threats – harm to self or others, running away

When one risk behavior as listed below is identified, watch for other concurrent risk behaviors which begin with experimentation, tend to cluster together and increase with age:

Unsafe sexual activity with risk of adolescent pregnancy and sexually transmitted diseases

Delinquent or antisocial behavior

Violence (with or without weapons)

Substance abuse

School failure

MANAGEMENT

Plan is dependent on the level of risk assessed and follows one of the following:

Reinforce and commend abstinence; include age appropriate anticipatory guidance

Focused counseling with emphasis on eliminating harmful health and behavioral consequences of substance abuse

Referral for appropriate treatment

BIBLIOGRAPHY

American College of Obstetricians and Gynecologists. *Tool Kit For Teen Care.* 2003. ACOG, Washington, DC

Dias PD. Adolescent substance abuse assessment in the office. *Pediatr Clin North Am* 2002;49:269–300

Elster A. *American Medical Association Guidelines for Adolescent Preventive Services (GAPS) Recommendations and Rationale.* Baltimore: Williams and Wilkins, 1994

24 Hirsutism

DEFINITION

Appearance of excessive coarse (terminal) male pattern hair growth in women; increase in distribution and quantity of terminal hair

KEY POINTS

In children may be the first sign of precocious puberty

In adolescents, may be idiopathic or an early sign of a tumor or pathologic condition of ovary or adrenal gland

Can be the first sign of impending virilization (clitoromegaly, temporal hair recession, deepening of the voice, changes in muscle pattern, breast atrophy)

Must be distinguished from hypertrichosis which refers to growth of hair in excess of normal while limited to normal distribution

DIFFERENTIAL DIAGNOSIS

Pediatric

Premature adrenarche 72%

Congenital adrenal hyperplasia 20%

Adrenocortical tumor 8%

Adolescent

- Idiopathic/genetic predisposition: 60–70% cases
- Ovarian causes:
  - Anovulation/polycystic ovarian syndrome (PCOS) (see Polycystic ovarian syndrome, Chapter 45)
  - Stromal hyperthecosis
  - Ovarian tumors
  - Enzyme deficiency (17-ketosteroid reductase)

- Adrenal causes:

    Congenital adrenal hyperplasia (CAH) (21-hydroxylase/11-beta-hydroxylase/3 beta-hydroxysteroid dehydrogenase deficiencies – see Ambiguous genitalia, Chapter 1)

- Cushing's syndrome – 2–5% of cases
- Tumors

Disorders of sexual differentiation (mixed gonadal dysgenesis)

Drug induced:

- Androgens, cyclosporin, danazol, diazoxide, glucocorticoids, minoxidil, phenytoin, testosterone, valproic acid

Other causes:

- Hypothyroidism/hyperprolactinemia
- Stress/anorexia

DIAGNOSIS

Task is to distinguish between idiopathic hirsutism and a pathologic condition

History

- Relation of hair growth to puberty and menses
- Gradual onset and progression – suggests idiopathic condition or chronic anovulation
- Rapid progression with deepening of the voice, severe acne – may indicate tumor
- Assess family history for PCOS/CAH
- Use of medications

Physical examination

Check weight, height

Look at hair pattern

- Evaluate for temporal balding, acne
- Quantify extent of hirsutism objectively with a Ferriman and Gallwey score (>8 is hirsute, see Figure 24-1)

Look at skin for acne and/or acanthosis nigricans (darkly pigmented skin at the nape of the neck, axilla, waist – associated with hyperinsulinemia/PCOS)

Look for stigmata of Cushing's disease (striae, moon facies)

Palpate for thyroid enlargement

Examine breasts for galactorrhea/atrophy

Evaluate for abdominal or pelvic masses

Laboratory evaluation

Check testosterone levels – elevation reflects ovarian androgen production

Dehydroepiandrosterone sulfate (DHEAS) – elevation reflects adrenal androgen production

IF patient not virilized: rule out other causes of androgen excess

- 1st screen for anovulation:

    Check prolactin, thyroid stimulating hormone (TSH), human choriogonadotropin (hCG) level

- Then check serum testosterone, DHEAS level

- 2nd screen for non-classical congenital adrenal hyperplasia:

    Obtain 7 a.m. 17-hydroxyprogesterone level

    > If > 300 ng/dl confirms CAH

    > If > 100 ng/dl need ACTH stimulation test

- 3rd screen for Cushing's syndrome:

    Obtain overnight dexamethasone suppression test

    > Give patient 1.0 mg dexamethasone @11p.m.

    > Draw fasting serum cortisol at 8:00 a.m.

    > Normal is < 5 ng/dl

IF patient virilized:

- Pediatric:

    Obtain DHEAS level:

    > With adrenarche usually > 40 µg/dl

    > If elevated, look for adrenal tumor or CAH

    Obtain serum testosterone:

    > If elevated, look for ovarian tumor

    > Obtain ultrasound

    Obtain 7 a.m. 17-hydroxyprogesterone (17-OHP) level

    > If > 100 ng/dl, need ACTH stimulation test (Draw baseline 17-OHP level then give 250 µg Cortrosyn IV then redraw 17-OHP level at 60 minutes)

    > If > 300 ng/dl, diagnostic of CAH

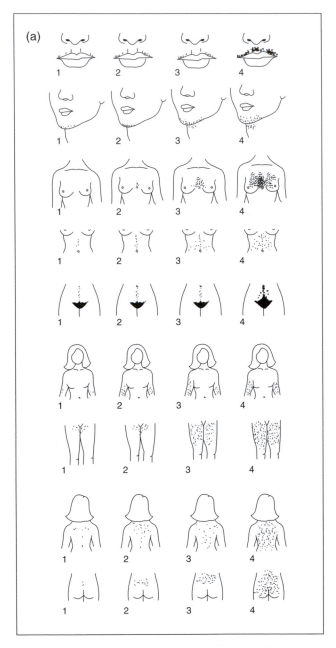

Figure 24-1a & b Hirsutism scoring sheet. The Ferriman and Gallwey system for scoring hirsutism. A score of 8 or more indicates hirsutism. Reproduced with permission from Hatch R, Rosenfield RL, Kim MH, *et al.* Hirsutism: implications, etiology, and management. *Am J Obstet Gynecol* 1981;149:815. © 1981 Mosby. Adapted from Ferriman D, Gallwey JD. Clinical assessment of body hair growth in women. *J Clin Endocrinol Metab* 1961;21:1440. Used with permission)

(b) *(Grade 0 at all sites indicates absence of terminal hair).*

Site	Grade	Definition
1. Upper lip	1	A few hairs at outer margin.
	2	A small moustache at outer margin.
	3	A moustache extending halfway from outer margin.
	4	A moustache extending to midline.
2. Chin	1	A few scattered hairs.
	2	Scattered hairs with small concentrations.
	3 & 4	Complete cover, light and heavy.
3. Chest	1	Circumareolar hairs.
	2	With mid-line hair in addition.
	3	Fusion of these areas, with three-quarter cover.
	4	Complete cover.
4. Upper back	1	A few scattered hairs.
	2	Rather more, still scattered.
	3 & 4	Complete cover, light and heavy.
5. Lower back	1	A sacral tuft of hair.
	2	With some lateral extension.
	3	Three-quarter cover.
	4	Complete cover
6. Upper abdomen	1	A few mid-line hairs
	2	Rather more, still mid-line.
	3 & 4	Half and full cover.
7. Lower abdomen	1	A few mid-line hairs
	2	A mid-line streak of hair.
	3	A mid-line band of hair.
	4	An inverted V-shaped growth.
8. Arm	1	Sparse growth affecting not more than a quarter of the limb surface.
	2	More than this; cover still incomplete.
	3 & 4	Complete cover, light and heavy.
9. Foream	1, 2, 3, 4	Complete cover of dorsal surface; 2 grades of light and 2 of heavy growth.
10. Thigh	1, 2, 3, 4	As for arm.
11. Leg	1, 2, 3, 4	As for arm.

- Adolescent:

  Obtain serum testosterone:

  Abnormal > 200 ng/dl suggests an ovarian androgen secreting tumor

  If > 150 ng/dl, then check pelvic ultrasound

  Obtain a serum (DHEAS):

  Abnormal > 700 µg/dl Suggests adrenal tumor

  Check CT or MRI of adrenals

  If negative, may need to do adrenocorticotropic hormone (ACTH) stimulation test to rule out CAH

MANAGEMENT

Treatment is targeted at the underlying cause

Eliminate causative factors

Optimize weight:

- Obesity is linked to anovulation, insulin resistance, lowered sex-hormone binding globulin levels

Manage hair:

- Bleaching
- Cutting or shaving
- Depilatory creams
- Electrolysis
- Laser epilation
- Plucking
- Waxing

Management of excess ovarian androgen production:

- Most commonly PCOS
- Use combination estrogen/progestin oral contraceptive pills (OCPs):

  Estrogen component increases sex-hormone binding globulin which binds circulating androgen thus decreasing androgen at hair follicle

  Progestin component inhibits luteinising hormone (LH) secretion, creating less ovarian androgen output.

- Use gonadotropin releasing hormone (GnRH) agonists in severe cases:

  Depot leuprolide (Lupron Depot®, TAP Pharmaceuticals, Inc., Lake Forest, IL) 3.75 mg IM monthly

  Will result in hypoestrogenism, may need to combine with estrogen or estrogen/progestin add-back (see Endometriosis, Chapter 18)

- If associated with insulin resistance: consider use of metformin (see Polycystic ovarian syndrome, Chapter 45)

  May need endocrinology consult for use

Management of excess adrenal androgen production:

- Little role for corticosteroid treatment unless adrenal enzyme deficiency

Management directed at hair follicle:

- Spironolactone:

  Decreases androgen production and blocks the androgen receptor at hair follicle

  May use in combination with oral contraceptives or alone

  Dose 100 mg po twice daily

  Does not alter hair already present but will decrease new growth

  May take up to 6 months to see response

  Need birth control with this if sexually active

If CAH, see Ambiguous genitalia (Chapter 1) for workup/management

If ovarian or adrenal tumor: needs surgical excision

BIBLIOGRAPHY

Emans SJ. Endocrine abnormalities associated with hirsutism. In Emans SJ, Laufer MR, Goldstein DP (eds). *Pediatric and Adolescent Gynecology*. 4th edn. Philadelphia: Lippincott-Raven Publishers, 1998;263–302

Jamieson MA. Hirsutism investigations – what is appropriate? *J Pediatr Adolesc Gynecol* 2001;14:95–7

Plouffe L. Disorders of excessive hair growth in the adolescent. *Obstet Gynecol Clin North Am* 2000;27:79–99

Rosenfield RL, Cara JF. Androgens and the adolescent girl. In Sanfilipppo JS, Muram D, Dewhurst J, Lee PA (eds). *Pediatric and Adolescent Gynecology*, 2nd edn. Philadelphia: WB Saunders, 2001:269–94

Schroeder B. Early diagnosis, presenting complaints, and management of hyperandrogenism in adolescents. *Curr Womens Health Rep* 2001;1:124–30

Street ME, Weber A, Camacho-Hubner C, *et al*. Girls with virilization in childhood: a diagnostic protocol for investigation. *J Clin Pathol* 1997;50:379–83

25 Hymenal anatomy (normal and abnormal)

Absence of the hymen has NEVER been reported in the literature; if absent, look for a reason

EXAMINATION

Please refer to the chapter on Gynecologic examination in the pediatric patient (Chapter 21) for a description on how to visualize the hymen

Prepubertal: use a moistened Dacron swab or a lubricated 5-mm pediatric feeding tube to best evaluate the perimeter of the hymen

Postpubertal non-sexually active: run hymen's perimeter using a moistened Q-tip to assess confluence; hormonal stimulation can fill in a laceration making any scars invisible and the hymenal perimeter appears uninterrupted; exam cannot be used to prove or disprove sexual penetration

PREPUBERTAL MORPHOLOGY

Annular (circumferential) see Figure 25-1: hymen extends completely around the circumference of the vaginal orifice

Crescentic (posterior rim) see Figure 25-2: hymen with anterior attachments at approximately the 11 o'clock and 1 o'clock positions with no hymenal tissue visible between the two attachments

Redundant see Figure 25-3: abundant hymenal tissue that tends to fold back upon itself or protrude

Fimbriated, see Figure 25-4: hymen with multiple projections or indentations along the edge

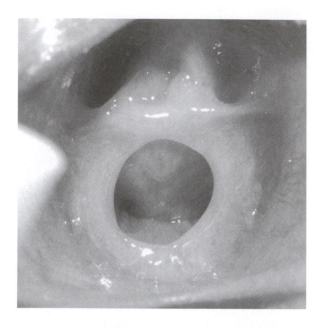

Figure 25-1 4-year-old African-American female; family concerns regarding child care center; no allegations of sexual contact; normal annular hymen. Reproduced with permission from: McCann JJ, Kerns DL. *The Anatomy of Child and Adolescent Sexual Abuse: A CD-ROM Atlas/Reference.* InterCorp, Inc., St. Louis, MO

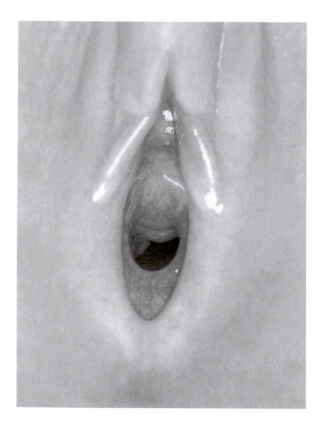

Figure 25-2 3-year-old Anglo female with crescentic hymen. Non-abuse study. Intravaginal longitudinal ridges. Labial separation, traction and prone knee–chest position. Reproduced with permission from: McCann JJ, Kerns DL. *The Anatomy of Child and Adolescent Sexual Abuse: A CD-ROM Atlas/Reference.* InterCorp, Inc., St. Louis, MO

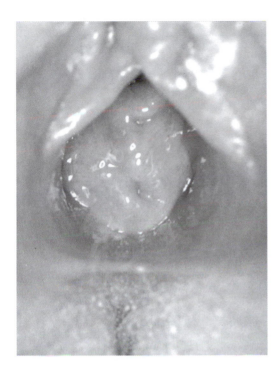

Figure 25-3   2-year-old Anglo female with a redundant hymen. Non-abuse study. Labial separation, traction and prone knee–chest position. Reproduced with permission from: McCann JJ, Kerns DL. *The Anatomy of Child and Adolescent Sexual Abuse: A CD-ROM Atlas/Reference.* InterCorp, Inc., St. Louis, MO

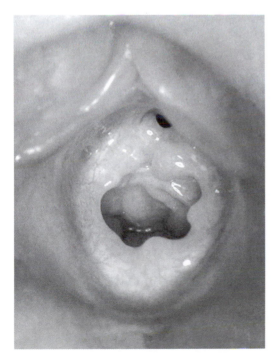

Figure 25-4   2-year-old Anglo female with a fimbriated hymen, a normal variation. Reproduced with permission from: McCann JJ, Kerns DL. *The Anatomy of Child and Adolescent Sexual Abuse: A CD-ROM Atlas/Reference.* InterCorp, Inc., St. Louis, MO

Table 25-1   Non-specific findings

Non-specific findings	McCann 1990	Berenson Heger 1991	Gardner 1992	Berenson Heger 1992	Hegar 2001
Number	86+	468	79	201	147
Periurethral/ perihymenal bands	50.6/16%	Frequent	14%	98%	91.8%
Longitudinal intravaginal ridges	90.2%	56		25%	93.8%
Hymenal tag	24.4%	13%	2%	3%	3.4%
Hymenal bump or mound	33.8%	< 1	11%	7%	34%
Linea vestibularis	15.7%		23%	4%	19%
Erythema	56%				48.9%
Change in vascularity	30.9%		44%	5%	37.4%
Labial adhesions	38.9%			17%	15.6%
Thickened hymenal rim	53.8%		Frequent		45.5%
Irregular hymenal rim	41.9%		9%		51.7%

+Supine with traction
Modified and used with permission from: Heger AH, Ticson L, Guerra L, *et al.* Appearance of the genitalia in girls selected for nonabuse: review of hymenal morphology and nonspecific findings. *J Pediatr Adoles Gynecol* 2002;15:27–35

NON-SPECIFIC PREPUBERTAL FINDINGS

See Table 25-1

MORPHOLOGY CHANGES WITH AGING TOWARDS PUBERTY

Increase in number of children with a crescentic configuration and **increasing** transverse and vertical diameters with aging between ages 1 and 3 and ages 3 and 9

Vertical diameters increase with BMI at ages 5 and 7

Number of mounds and intravaginal ridges increased with aging but frequently associated with preexisting ridges

No significant changes with number of tags, vestibular bands, notches, periurethral bands or external ridges

At menarche, hymen has progressed from crescentic to fimbriated, reddened and thick morphology

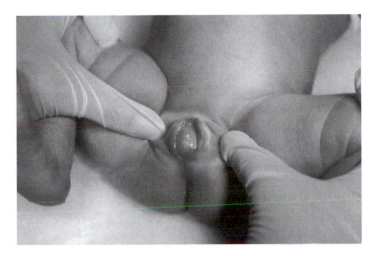

Figure 25-5   An imperforate hymen in a newborn girl

INDICATIONS OF SEXUAL ABUSE*

Result from penetrative injuries unless proven otherwise (still very rare, only seen if exam within 72 hours or if bleeding at time of injury)

Acute laceration or ecchymosis of the hymen

Absence of hymenal tissue in the posterior half

Healed hymenal transection or complete cleft

At least 1 mm of hymenal tissue should be present at the 6 o'clock position between the hymenal rim and vaginal floor in prepubertal girls without a history of abuse or trauma

*Transhymenal diameter is no longer used as an indicator of abuse

CONGENITAL ABNORMALITIES

Hymen: imperforate

Newborn

With mucocolpos (see Figure 25-5)

If diagnosed before leaving the hospital: feed bottle for comfort, use a needle point bovie to open, place stay suture of 4-0 Vicryl at 6 o'clock position

If diagnosed after leaving the hospital: mucocolpos should subside within one month; would wait to correct until significant pubertal development unless symptoms of gastrointestinal or urinary obstruction

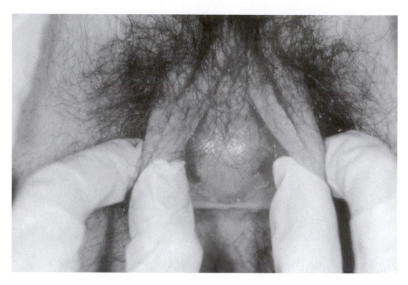

Figure 25-6   Imperforate hymen and hematocolpos in an adolescent girl

Without mucocolpos

> Wait until significant pubertal development to correct; procedure as with adolescent

Adolescent

(See Figure 25-6)

Presenting symptoms:

> Found incidentally with well-child exam
>
> Found symptomatic: cyclic abdominal pain, urinary retention

Physical examination:

> Asymptomatic: hard to assess, try probing with a feeding tube or calgi swab if patient tolerates. If unable to tolerate follow with serial exams or ultrasound as Tanner staging progresses
>
> Symptomatic: presents with hematocolpos, a bulging bluish mass at the introitus; if unclear diagnosis, try rectal exam; if still unclear, use ultrasound or MRI to distinguish from cervical agenesis, transverse vaginal septum or agenesis of the lower third of the vagina (see Vaginal tract abnormalities, Chapter 66)

Treatment:

> If unable to repair immediately, suppress the ovaries with continuous oral contraceptives or GnRH agonist and narcotic analgesia until suppression is completed

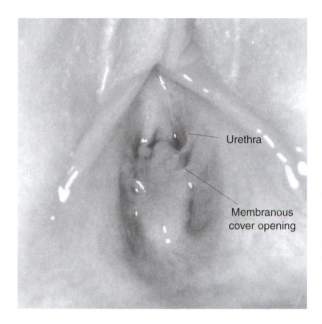

Urethra

Membranous
cover opening

Figure 25-7   18-month-old with a microperforate hymenal orifice. Multiple periurethral and perihymenal bands. Reproduced with permission from: McCann JJ, Kerns DL. *The Anatomy of Child and Adolescent Sexual Abuse: A CD-ROM Atlas/Reference.* InterCorp, Inc., St. Louis, MO

Repair:

- General anesthesia
- Place indwelling urethral catheter to avoid injury secondary to distortion
- Make cruciate incision with needlepoint bovie
- Use eye protection as fluid may be under pressure
- Have two suction catheter sets as one may become obstructed
- After draining, excise remainder of excess hymenal tissue
- Normal size is calibrated to allow placement of Huffman speculum
- Vaginal mucosa can be sutured to hymenal ring to prevent regression and stenosis with interrupted 4-0 Vicryl sutures
- Postoperative care of 48 hours of ice packs prn comfort followed by sitz baths until sutures healed. Use of estrogen cream to the area on a daily basis for a week may enhance healing

Hymen: microperforate

(See Figure 25-7)

Definition:

Hymenal tissue completely covers the vaginal opening with microperforate opening at the 12 o'clock position just below the periurethral tissue

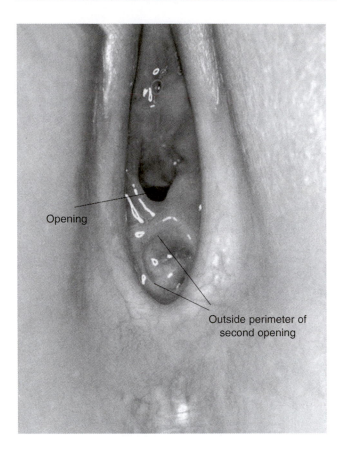

Opening

Outside perimeter of
second opening

Figure 25-8   3-year-old Anglo female with a midline hymenal defect; cribriform hymen, a congenital variation. Reproduced with permission from: McCann JJ, Kerns DL. *The Anatomy of Child and Adolescent Sexual Abuse: A CD-ROM Atlas/Reference.* InterCorp, Inc., St. Louis, MO

Treatment:

Remove only if requested to enhance tampon use or permit sexual activity or noted to have incomplete emptying of menses or vaginal discharge

Perform removal under general anesthesia. Resect with a needle point bovie under general anesthesia. Interrupted 4-0 Vicryl suture as needed for hemostasis. Postoperative care as with imperforate hymen

Final result should be similar to that recommended for adolescent imperforate hymen

Hymen: cribriform

(See Figure 25-8)

Definition:

Hymen stretches completely across the vaginal opening but has varied microperforate openings throughout

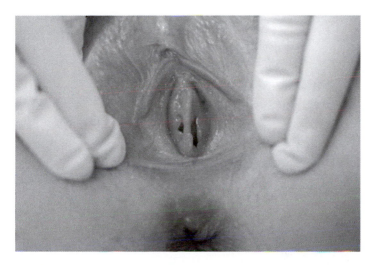

Figure 25-9   Septated hymen

Treatment:

Remove only if requested to enhance tampon use or permit sexual activity or noted to have incomplete emptying of menses or vaginal discharge

Perform removal under general anesthesia. Resect with a needle point bovie under general anesthesia. Interrupted 4-0 Vicryl suture as needed for hemostasis. Postoperative care as with imperforate hymen

Final result should be similar to that recommended for adolescent imperforate hymen

Hymen: septum

(See Figure 25-9)

Definition:

Bands of tissue that bisect the orifice, creating two or more openings

Treatment:

Remove only if requested to enhance tampon use or permit sexual activity

If patient cooperative and septum not too thick, tie a 3-0 chromic suture around the middle and septum should necrose at suture line

If patient not cooperative or septum too thick, perform removal under general anesthesia. Tie an absorbable suture, i.e. 4-0 chromic around each base and remove middle with needle point bovie

Postoperative care as with imperforate hymen

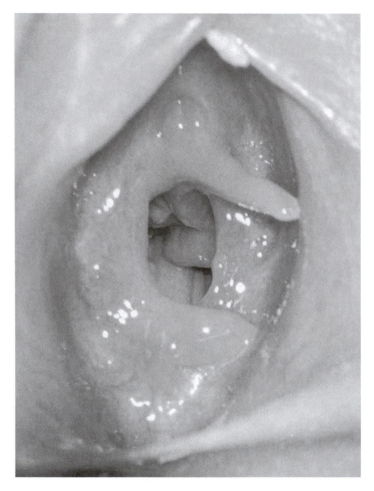

Figure 25-10   10-month-old Anglo female with a hymenal tag that appears to be an extension of a posterior vaginal column. Reproduced with permission from: McCann JJ, Kerns DL. *The Anatomy of Child and Adolescent Sexual Abuse: A CD-ROM Atlas/Reference.* InterCorp, Inc., St. Louis, MO

Hymen: tags

(See Figure 25-10)

Treatment:

Remove only if symptomatic

If thin and child motivated, tie absorbable suture tightly around base and allow to necrose off

If too thick or child prefers, perform removal under general anesthesia; needle point bovie, suture base with 4-0 Vicryl absorbable suture; postoperative care as with imperforate hymen

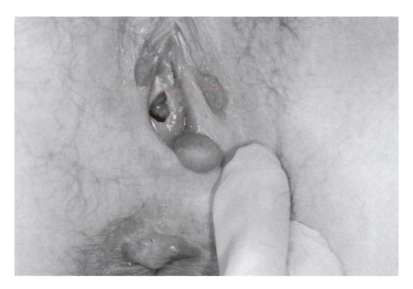

Figure 25-11   Hymenal cyst

Hymen: cyst

(See Figure 25-11)

Treatment:

Remove only if symptomatic

Perform removal under general anesthesia. Use a needle point bovie under anesthesia, suture hymenal base with absorbable suture, i.e. 4-0 Vicryl

Postoperative care as with imperforate hymen

BIBLIOGRAPHY

Berenson AB, Grady JJ. A longitudinal study of hymenal development from 3–9 years of age. *J Pediatr* 2002:140;600–7

Heger AH, Ticson L, Guerra L, *et al*. Appearance of the genitalia in girls selected for nonabuse: review of hymenal morphology and nonspecific findings. *J Pediatr Adoles Gynecol* 2002;15:27–35

26 Labial abscess

Labial abscesses originate in the skin and may result from some type of trauma

Typically seen in prepubertal or immunosuppressed (including diabetic) adolescent

Organism is usually skin flora: *Staphylococcus* or *Streptococcus*

Glandular abscesses most commonly in the Bartholin's glands but can arise from the Gartner's or Skene's glands

Typically seen in menstruating female

Organisms range from *Chlamydia* and/or gonorrhea to anaerobes

DIAGNOSIS

History

Localized edema, erythema and pain of the labia

History of previous labial abscess

Associated symptoms of fever, discomfort or drainage

Physical examination

Visual signs of swelling, redness and tenderness on a unilateral portion of the labia

+/– Fever

+/– Discharge from mass

MANAGEMENT

Child

If cooperative: ultrasound guided needle aspiration prior to treatment; Pre-aspiration application of EMLA® cream to skin of area to be probed (see EMLA® use, Chapter 17); send for aerobic and anaerobic culture with Gram stain

If uncooperative, without systemic symptoms (i.e. sepsis), admit for IV antibiotics; if failing treatment without systemic symptoms, ultrasound guided needle aspiration with EMLA® and/or IV sedation and send for culture as above

Warm compresses or sitz baths 3–4x a day

Antibiotics for 7–10 days:

- Dicloxacillin 12–25 mg/kg/day po divided qid
- Cephalexin 25–50 mg/kg/day po divided qid
- If there is no improvement within 24 h or in the presence of a fever over 101°F (38.3°C) or elevated white blood cell count or if the patient is immunocompromised, intravenous medication should be initiated with the same medications until organism identified

Analgesia:

NSAIDs (20 mg/kg/24 h q 8 h), Tylenol (10–15 mg/kg/dose q 4–6 h) with codeine (0.5–1.0 mg/kg/dose q 4–6 h) or Tylenol with oxycodone (0.5–0.15 mg/kg/dose q 4 h)

Antipyretic for temperature greater than or equal to 100°F (37.8°C):

Tylenol or NSAID

Follow-up twice weekly:

Watch for recurrence. May need I&D

I&D:

Should be done if no improvement within 48 h or with worsening signs or symptoms

Should be done with sedation

Culture for aerobic and anaerobic organisms

Pack with plain Nugauze

Sitz bath qid

Change packing once daily, may need sedation

Complications:

Recurrent infections: check for diabetes mellitus, immunosupression, and chronic *Staphylococcus* carrier (aerobic C&S swab of nares)

Scarring

Adolescent

Labial abscess:

Treat as above. Screen for diabetes mellitus. If sexually active, screen for sexually transmitted diseases and pregnancy

Bartholin's gland abscess: see Bartholin's abscess (Chapter 3)

27 Labial adhesions (labial agglutination)

KEY POINTS

Usually an asymptomatic incidental finding with thin, flat, pale membranous line between labia minora starting at the posterior fourchette and ending just below the clitoral hood

Occasionally diagnosed when symptoms of urinary retention, urinary tract infection or vulvovaginitis are being evaluated

Peak incidence 13–23 months of age

Typically resolves with endogenous estrogen at puberty

Adhesions that occur after puberty are customarily associated with previous surgical procedures or vulvar trauma

DIFFERENTIAL DIAGNOSIS

Urogenital sinus

Congenital absence of vagina

Transverse vaginal septum

Imperforate hymen

MANAGEMENT

Asymptomatic: no treatment unless persist into puberty

Symptomatic – frequent urinary tract infections, difficulty with urination, persistence into puberty:

Topical estrogen cream applied bid up to 6 weeks: place labia on traction to visualize the midline adhesion and massage a very small amount of cream into the adhesion

If adhesion not open after 6 weeks, apply emollient, i.e. A&D in same fashion for next 2 weeks, then return to estrogen for 6 weeks. If still not open after this may repeat process (if progressively opening) or may surgically open (see below)

Avoid possible irritants (i.e. soap, bubblebaths) (see Pamphlet listed below)

Warn parents that breast budding can occur with topical estrogen, to substitute A&D or other emollient until budding ceases

Once adhesion is open place a small amount of estrogen cream or A&D between the labia for several weeks

Warn parents and patient that resolution may take several courses of treatment; agglutination can recur until menstruation starts

Symptomatic – urinary retention:

Use EMLA® cream (see EMLA® Use, Chapter 17) or lidocaine jelly 2%

IV sedation should be utilized in children over 18 months just prior to separation

Separate by placing a moistened Q-tip inside or on top of the adhesion and opening with gentle pressure

After opening use estrogen cream daily for 6 weeks between labia minora to prevent recurrence

Check urine for infection

Avoid possible irritants (i.e. soap, bubblebaths (see Pamphlet listed below)

Warn parents and patients that agglutination can recur until menstruation starts

PAMPHLET

North American Society for Pediatric and Adolescent Gynecology. *Pediatric Vulvovaginitis*. Telephone 215-955-6331

28 Labial asymmetry/ hypertrophy

KEY POINTS

Asymmetry often first noted at menarche

This is not generally a pathologic condition

Usually is asymptomatic/requires no treatment

DEFINITION

Large labia minora projecting beyond the labia majora

When maximal distance between base and edge is > 4 cm

Enlargement may be unilateral (asymmetric) or bilateral

ETIOLOGY

Congenital/hereditary

Acquired

Chronic irritation

Recurrent dermatitis (e.g. secondary to urinary incontinence)

Trauma

Childbirth

Exogenous androgenic hormonal influence

Infection

Idiopathic

DIAGNOSIS

History

Symptoms

> Local irritation

> Pain/discomfort with tight clothing

> Discomfort in walking or sitting

> Problems with hygiene during menses or after bowel movements

> Sexual self-consciousness

> Personal/family history of:

> Skin disorders

> Inflammatory bowel disease

Physical examination

Height/weight (plot on growth curves) (See Obesity, Chapter 35)

> Patients with chronic disease, inflammatory bowel disease may have limited growth

Vulvar assessment

> Assess for labial mass vs hypertrophy

> Assess for other genital abnormalities that could account for irritation

> - Vulvar varicosities
> - Skin conditions
> - Yeast infections
> - Vulvar manifestations for Crohn's disease

> Measure distance between base and edge of labia

MANAGEMENT

IF maximal distance between base and edge < 4 cm:

> No treatment necessary

> Provide reassurance, variation in size is normal and remainder of examination is normal

IF maximal distance between base and edge of labia is > 4 cm and patient is symptomatic:

Offer labia minoral reduction:

- W- or V-shaped wedge reduction of enlarged labia with reapproximation of remaining tissue *or*
- Deepithelialized reduction labioplasty

    Reduces significantly enlarged, asymmetrical or distended interior labia

Indication for surgery: Size alone (> 4 cm) **not** an indication unless accompanied by:

Aesthetic concerns

Discomfort in clothing

Discomfort with exercise

Entry dyspareunia

Hygienic reasons

Chronic irritation

Need to make urinary self-catheterization easier

Note: If patient is under age 18, patient and parents should be counselled prior to surgery that labial growth may continue after surgery

BIBLIOGRAPHY

Alter GJ. A new technique for aesthetic labia minora reduction. *Ann Plast Surg* 1998;40:287–90

Choi HY, Kim KT. A new method for aesthetic reduction of labia minora (the deepithelialized reduction labioplasty). *Plas Reconstr Surg* 2000;105:419–22

Maas S, Hage JJ. Functional and aesthetic labia minora reduction. *Plas Reconstr Surg* 2000;105:1453–6

Rouzier, R, Louis-Sylvestre C, Paniel BJ, Bassam H. Hypertrophy of labia minora: Experience with 163 reductions. *Am J Obstet Gynecol* 2000;182:35–40

Werlin SL, Esterly NB, Oechler H. Crohn's disease presenting as unilateral labial hypertrophy. *J Am Acad Dermatol* 1992;27:893–5

29 Labial/vulvar mass

Cysts are common, most are congenital and appear at birth or with hormonal stimulation at adolescence

Tumors are uncommon and most are benign

DIFFERENTIAL DIAGNOSIS

Congenital or acquired hernia (often contain the ovary)

Gonadal remnant

Embryonic remnant:

- Paraurethral cyst
- Hymenal cyst
- Mesonephric (Gartner duct) cyst
- Canal of Nuck cyst
    Peritoneum along round ligament filled with fluid
- Bartholin's duct cyst
    Posterior labia majora location

Mesenchymal tumors

- Striated muscle: Rhabdomyoma
- Fat: Lipoma
- Fibrous tissue: Fibroma
- Lymphatics: Lymphangioma
- Neural tissue: Granular cell tumor
                            Neurofibromatosis
- Vascular tissue: Hemangioma

Suppurative conditions:

- Hidradenitis suppuritiva

Malignant tumors:

- Embryonal rhabdomyosarcoma (sarcoma botryoides)

    Usually vaginal in origin

- Endodermal sinus tumor
- Primitive neuroectodermal tumors (PNET)
- Squamous cell carcinoma
- Malignant melanoma

Precocious puberty – will likely have other secondary sexual characteristics

Congenital adrenal hyperplasia (CAH) – will likely have other hormonal changes, ie. clitoromegaly, advanced growth, hirsutism

Vulvar varicosities

Rare causes

- Crohn's disease
- Hamartoma

EVALUATION

History

- Onset and duration of symptomatic mass
- Pain/tenderness
- Past history:

    Neurofibromatosis

    Inflammatory bowel disease

- Review of symptoms:

    Gastrointestinal complaints (abdominal pain/diarrhea) – to rule out Crohn's disease

Physical examination

- Examine entire skin surface/buccal mucosa for lesions

    Look for café-au-lait macules indicating neurofibromatosis

- Examine vulva for location, extent and quality of mass

    Look at color(s), measure size, note fluctuance or tenderness

Laboratory/testing

- If suspect precocious puberty:

    Follicle stimulating hormone, estradiol levels (diagnosis likely if either elevated)

- If genitalia ambiguous:

    Rule out CAH with 7 a.m. 17-hydroxyprogesterone level, dehydroepiandrosterone sulfate level

- Karyotype and testosterone level:

    Determine if mass of testicular origin

- Use perineal/pelvic ultrasound to:

    Diagnose hernia, evaluate mass for peripheral follicles of an ovary and/or determine solid/cystic nature of mass and to document internal anatomy ruling out concomitant pelvic tumors

    Note: Sliding indirect inguinal hernias may require more than a single examination to diagnose

- MRI may help further define large masses

MANAGEMENT

Based on etiology:

Hidradenitis suppurativa

- Suppurative condition of apocrine glands resulting in follicular occlusion and multiple furuncles and ultimately cysts and draining fistulous tracts
- Can involve the breasts, axilla and other intertriginous areas as well
- Early lesions: subepithelial swellings that appear firm and/or fluctuant
- Treatment: Local care with warm baths

    Non-irritating loose clothing

    Oral antibiotics (doxycycline) and topical antiseptics (Phisoderm) with oral contraceptive pills and anti-androgens (spironolactone)

    Severe cases: surgical excision but is disfiguring and does not prevent recurrence

Lymphangioma

Common with congenital lymphedema of lower extremities

No treatment unless symptomatic

Leiomyoma and lipoma

  No intervention unless symptomatic

Neurofibromas

  Uncommon in children

  May be the earliest clinical manifestation of neurofibromatosis

  Suspect in the presence of multiple café-au-lait spots

  Rarely solitary

  Vaginoscopy/cystoscopy may reveal presence of neurofibromas in the vagina or bladder

  Rarely malignant

Granular cell tumor

  Schwann cell origin

  Excision is curative

Malignant neoplasms

  Squamous cell carcinoma

  - Reported but uncommon in adolescents
  - Presents as a raised lesion which can be ulcerated and confused with an infectious process
  - Biopsy all non-healing ulcers

  Sarcoma botryoides (embryonal rhabdomyosarcoma)

  - Large lesion that may present as 'flesh colored grapes'
  - Treatment is now multimodal involving chemotherapy, radiation and surgery

  Endodermal sinus tumors

  - Very rare
  - Alpha-fetoprotein levels have been reported to be normal
  - Poor prognosis

  Malignant melanoma

  - Rarely reported

  In some cases, may be able to use topical EMLA® (see EMLA® use, Chapter 17) then infiltrate with lidocaine to do an in-office incisional biopsy; in others may need surgical excision

Hernias require surgical repair to prevent prolapse of the ovary into hernia

Hemangiomas: see Hemangioma of vulva (Chapter 22)

When etiology uncertain, excision of mass is indicated

BIBLIOGRAPHY

Lowry DLB, Guido RS. The vulvar mass in the prepubertal child. *J Pediatr Adolesc Gynecol* 2000;13:75–8

Munden M, McEniff N, Mulvihill D. Sonographic investigation of female infants with inguinal masses. *Clin Radiol* 1995;50:696–8

Scherr GR, D'Ablaing G, Ouzounizn JG. Peripheral primitive neuroectodermal tumor of the vulva. *Gynecol Oncol* 1994;54:254–8

Werlin SL, Esterly NB, Oechler H. Crohn's disease presenting as unilateral labial hypertrophy. *J Am Acad Dermatol* 1992;27:893–5

30 Lichen sclerosus

DEFINITION

Chronic skin disorder of unknown cause that most commonly occurs in adult women. 10–15% cases arise in childhood and affect genitalia

DIAGNOSIS

Classic figure of eight distribution of white parchment-like epithelium around the clitoris, labia minora, perineal body and anus

May have subepithelial hemorrhages and superficial ulcerations

Common presenting complaints include pruritis, pain, dysuria, hematuria and constipation

Can be mistaken for sexual abuse

May need biopsy to confirm, but typical appearance is usually diagnostic

MANAGEMENT

Topical clobetasol proprionate (Temovate) ointment 0.05% applied sparingly to affected areas bid after bathing and good drying for 2–4 weeks then tapered to a less potent steroid ointment (i.e. Cutivate, Glaxo Wellcome, Inc., Research Triangle Park, NC; then to Aclovate, Glaxo Wellcome, Inc., Research Triangle Park, NC; Synalar, Medicis, The Dermatology Co., Scottsdale, AZ; hydrocortisone 0.2%) for 2 weeks; then to an OTC steroid ointment for 2 weeks and then off:

If no improvement, culture for yeast and aerobic bacteria and treat accordingly

Persistent use of ultrapotent steroids can cause epithelial atrophy and telengiectasia

After the initial flare is controlled, close observation for 6–12 months to monitor for recurrences. If missed can lead to significant labial, periclitoral and clitoral hood scarring

Most cases resolve with puberty

BIBLIOGRAPHY

Ridley CM. Dermatologic conditions of the vulva. In Sanfilippo JS, Muram DM, Dewhurst J, Lee PA, eds. *Pediatric and Adolescent Gynecology*, 2nd edn. Philadelphia, PA: WB Saunders, 2001:230–2

31 Menstruation

NORMAL

First period or menarche occurs on average at 12.43 years of age

Menarche typically occurs about 2 years after thelarche (breast budding) (range 1–3 years)

Almost everyone has had menarche by age 16

Menstrual cycles occur every 21–45 days after menarche

Menses last 3–5 days with range of 2–7 days

Menses become regular after 2–2.5 years

While early cycles are anovulatory the pattern is regularly irregular, not erratic

Therefore:

- Evaluate for specific causes of amenorrhea in girls with cycles > 90 days (e.g. pregnancy, eating disorders, hypothalamic amenorrhea)

ABNORMAL

DEFINITIONS

Amenorrhea: absence of menses (for evaluation see Amenorrhea, Chapter 2)

Primary amenorrhea:	No menses by age 14 in absence of secondary sexual characteristics *or*
	No menses by 2 years after completing sexual development *or*
	No menses by age 16 regardless of secondary sexual characteristics
Secondary amenorrhea:	No menses for 3–6 months in previously menstruating women

| Dysfunctional uterine bleeding: | Prolonged excessive menstrual bleeding associated with irregular periods, usually due to anovulation or immaturity of reproductive axis in adolescents within 2 years of menarche (For evaluation see Dysfunctional uterine bleeding, Chapter 13) |

Variations in frequency:

Polymenorrhea:	Frequent regular or irregular bleeding at < 21 day intervals
Oligomenorrhea:	Infrequent irregular bleeding at > 35 day intervals
Irregular menses:	Bleeding at varying intervals, > 21 days but < 35 day intervals

Variation in amount and duration:

Metrorrhagia:	Intermenstrual irregular bleeding between regular periods
Menorrhagia:	Regular/excessive amount, increased duration of uterine bleeding
Menometrorrhagia:	Frequent irregular, excessive, and prolonged episodes of uterine bleeding > 7 days in duration

32 Menstrual management of the mentally limited patient

KEY POINTS

Mentally limited patients may have difficulty with menstrual hygiene and understanding the process of menstruation; therefore, caretakers of these patients may request assistance with menstrual management issues

EVALUATION

History

Assessment of patient's disability, prognosis for independent living, continence patterns, cognitive function, susceptibility for abuse:

  If possible, both with parent and alone

  Description of menstrual patterns, premenstrual and menstrual behaviors

  Associated symptoms i.e. dysmenorrhea, bowel and urinary changes

Complete: medical, surgical, family and symptom review history

Physical examination

Assess thyroid, breast, abdomen, extremities, heart and lungs, external genitalia +/− speculum and bimanual exam

Laboratory tests

With history of menorrhagia – complete blood count with platelets, PT/PTT; Von Willebrand's Factor (VWF) Panel (VWF antigen, factor VIII, ristocetin cofactor activity levels) (see Dysfunctional uterine bleeding, Chapter 13)

IF strong family history of venous thromboembolic disease: thrombophilia work-up (see Contraception, Chapter 11)

Pregnancy test if missed just one menses

Pregnancy test, follicle stimulating hormone (FSH), thyroid stimulating hormone (TSH), prolactin, total and % free testosterone if missed menses more than 3 months or irregular

Transabdominal ultrasound if unable to perform pelvic exam

MANAGEMENT

If still in diapers, would treat symptoms:

Dysmenorrhea with non-steroidal antiinflammatory drugs, (see Dysmenorrhea, Chapter 14) – naproxen comes as an elixir 125 mg/tsp

Menstrual dysfunction (see Menstruation, Chapter 31; Dysfunctional uterine bleeding, Chapter 13)

If not in diapers but patient plays with body excrement and/or body fluids and unable to cognitively understand the consequences:

Medical management: (see Contraception, Chapter 11 for any contraindications for a particular method and for instructions how to use):

(1) Combination oral contraceptives:

- Goal is to induce predictable, manageable light menses
- Use lowest estrogen dose possible

(2) DepoProvera®:

- Goal is to suppress menses
- 150 mg IM per month × 3 and possibly until amenorrheic then every 8 weeks × 2 then every 10 weeks × 2 then every 12 weeks
- Emphasize calcium supplementation: 1300–1600 mg/day (see Osteoporosis, Chapter 38)
- Emphasize weight-bearing exercise
- Counsel family about increased appetite and hence increased weight and bone loss
- Check bone density after one year of amenorrhea. Given that there is no pediatric standard for bone density, consider obtaining a baseline bone density prior to treatment. Inform patient and family insurance may not cover bone density screening in the absence of a diagnosis of osteoporosis

(3) Lupron Depot®:

- Use 3.75 mg IM every 28 days for 2–3 months to induce amenorrhea then switch to DepoProvera® 150 mg IM every 12 weeks

- Warn family regarding potential for large withdrawal bleed 2–3 weeks after the first injection

Surgical mangement:

Should not and cannot be undertaken as initial treatment

Options include: endometrial ablation with tubal ligation, or hysterectomy; in many states, court approval is required for a minor to have such a procedure

If menstrual disorder:

Would treat as any other adolescent in terms of menstrual disorders and contraception. See Menstruation (Chapter 31), Dysfunctional uterine bleeding (Chapter 13), Contraception (Chapter 11), Sexual activity (Chapter 55)

BIBLIOGRAPHY

Quint EH. The conservative management of abnormal bleeding in teenagers with developmental disabilities. *J Pediatr Adolesc Gynecol* 2003;16:54–6

Quint EH. Gynecological care for teenagers with disabilities (Review). *J Pediatr Adolesc Gynecol* 2003;16:115–7

Zurawin RK, Paransky OI. The role of surgical techniques in the treatment of menstrual problems and as contraception in adolescents with disabilities. *J Pedratr Adolesc Gynecol* 2003;16:51–4

33 Molluscum contagiosum

DEFINITION

A common cutaneous viral infection caused by a poxvirus that results in classic firm, waxy, dome-shaped umbilicated lesions of the epidermis that is spread by skin-to-skin contact with an infected person or material (e.g. clothing, towel)

KEY POINTS

Highly transmissible

Usually a self-limited infection in children

In immunodeficient patients can be severely disfiguring and intractable

Secondary bacterial infection is a common complication

DIFFERENTIAL DIAGNOSIS

Genital warts

Dermatitis, atopic

Herpes simplex

Herpes zoster

DIAGNOSIS

History

Single or multiple discrete, painless papules (2–6 mm diameter) with a central depression

Lesions can be anywhere on the body, more likely to be on the extremities and therefore on the vulva

May spontaneously resolve

May have super infection

Lack of systemic symptoms

Patient/parent may recall contact with infected person – incubation period of about 2–6 weeks

For lesions limited to the vulva, ask about sexual abuse/consensual sexual contact

Physical examination

Well-defined, painless, pearly- or flesh-colored dome-shaped papules, 2–6 mm in diameter with central umbilication, may occur anywhere on the body, typically trunk, upper extremity, face and genitalia

Beneath the umbilicated center is a white cordlike core

In immunocompromized patients, lesions are more widespread and 10–15 mm in diameter

In sexually active teen, check for other sexually transmitted diseases (chlamydia and gonorrhea)

Laboratory tests

Diagnosis usually clinical due to classic appearance

Can confirm with biopsy, send for hematoxylin and eosin (H & E) staining

MANAGEMENT

Disease is usually self-limited, may not need treatment

Immunocompetent patient

Mainstay of therapy is destruction of the lesions

Initiate treatment with topical therapy with imiquimod: an immune response modifier (Not FDA approved for use in children but recommended/reported in medical literature)

- Imiquimod 5% cream:

    Adolescent: Apply small amount to cover the lesion and rub into lesion at bedtime, wash off in the morning. Repeat 3 × week for 6 weeks (may use up to 9–12 weeks). Reevaluate every 2–3 weeks for response

Pediatric/early adolescent: (use once/week to twice/week)

Can cause significant erosion/irritation to vulvar epithelium/may be more severe in prepubertal child, may wish to apply test dose with a cotton-tipped swab to one lesion first week of therapy and then reevaluate before extending area of treatment

Decrease frequency of use if severe irritation occurs

Erythema at lesion indicates medicine is working

If desire immediate removal or have only a few lesions:

- Curettage or enucleate the central plug of lesion:

    May apply EMLA® cream (see EMLA® use, Chapter 17) before curettage

Alternative destructive therapy:

- Cantharidin: a protein phosphatase inhibitor

    (Cantharidin preparations are banned by the FDA in the US however pure cantharidin and flexible collodion can be purchased by Delasco in the premeasured amounts to be combined for use to treat, see Epstein reference)

    Adult (adolescent)/pediatric dose: Apply sparingly with a wooden toothpick or the blunt wooden end of a cotton tipped applicator to each lesion, avoiding contact with normal skin. Have patient sit still and wait 5 minutes to allow cantharidin to completely dry. Maximum treatment to 20 lesions per visit

    Wash off in 4–6 hours or sooner if severe burning/irritation or vesiculation noted

    Repeat follow-up/therapy 2 to 4 weeks

    Can cause significant local irritation with blister; initially try on one or two lesions to test patient's sensitivity

Alternative medical treatments:

- Antihistamines (H2 blockers)

    Cimetidine (Tagamet®): mechanism of action not understood

    Adult (adolescent > 45 kg) dose: 300 mg po qid

    Pediatric dose: 30–40 mg/kg/day po divided qid

Immunocompromised patient

Seek assistance from pediatric dermatology with use of antiviral drugs

Cidofovir (Vistide®): Selective inhibitor of viral DNA

Successful in immunocompromised patients

Adult (adolescent > 45 kg) dose:	5 mg/kg IV over 1 hour, once q 2 weeks
Pediatric dose:	Same dose as adult

Topical use of 1% or 3% preparation applied to lesion then occluded with tape once daily for 5 days/weeks for 8 weeks

IV use is associated with:

Renal toxicity*, must prehydrate with normal saline and monitor renal function

Granulocytopenia may occur*

Ritonavir(Norvir®):	HIV protease inhibitor
Adult dose:	300–600 mg bid with meals
Pediatric dose:	> 16 years: initially 250 mg/m² bid

Titrate up to 400 mg/m² bid

< 16 years: not established

*Note: many drug interactions

Prognosis

Disease is usually self-limited

Lesions can persist for 2 weeks to 4 years

Recurrences can occur in up to 35% patients

When immunocompromised or HIV infected, disease is generalized

Instruct parent to watch for superinfection, antibiotic treatment to cover *Staphylococcus epidermidis* and *Streptococcus* species is required if super infection does occur

BIBLIOGRAPHY

Bretz S. Molluscum Contagiosum. Emedicine, June 11, 2002. www.emedicine.com/ emerg/topic 317.htm

Dohil M, Prendiville JS. Treatment of molluscum contagiosum with oral cimetidine: clinical experience in 13 patients. *Pediatr Dermatol* 1996; 13:310–12

Epstein E. Cantharidin therapy for molluscum contagiosum in children. *J Am Acad Dermatol* 2001;45:638

Liota E, Smith K, Buckley R, *et al*. Imiquimod therapy for molluscum contagiosum. *J Cutaneous Med Surg* 2000;4:76–82

Silverberg NB, Sidbury R, Mancini AJ. Childhood molluscum contagiosum: experience with cantharidin therapy in 300 patients. *J Am Acad Dermatol* 2000; 43:503–7

Toro JR, Wood LV, Patel NK, *et al*. Topical cidofovir: a novel treatment for recalcitrant molluscum contagiosum in children infected with human immunodeficiency virus 1. *Arch Dermatol* 2000;136:983–5

34 Nipple discharge

Not representative of a single problem

Could be several different conditions

Typically benign condition/rarely associated with malignancy

DIAGNOSIS

Helpful to classify discharge on color/type:

Endocrine/milky

Represents galactorrhea

- Usually respond to elevated prolactin production:

  Following pregnancy/abortion

  Drug induced

  Prolactin-secreting tumor of pituitary

  Idiopathic

- Etiology:

  Neurogenic

  Pituitary

  Drug induced

  Idiopathic

  Persistent breast stimulation (e.g. rubbing of nipple on bra seam)

  Hypothyroidism

  Pregnancy-related

- History: Persistent nipple stimulation

  Use of medications/drugs:

Amitriptyline	Meprobamate
Amphetamines	Methyldopa
Androgens	Metoclopramide
Anesthetics	Monoamine oxidase inhibitors
Chlorpromazine	Narcotics
Cimetidine	Opiates
Domperidone	Phenothiazines
Estrogens	Prostaglandins
Fluphenazine	Reserpine
Haloperidol	Spironolactone

- Physical: Evaluate for presence of goiter

  Visual field impairment

  Chest wall deformity

  Pubertal aberration

  Attempt to express fluid from breasts

  Unilateral typically not systemic cause

- Laboratory: Prolactin (PRL), thyroid stimulating hormone (TSH) levels

  Prolactin > 100 ng/ml requires MRI of pituitary

  If hypothyroid, PRL will also be increased

  Treat hypothyroidism with replacement

  Follow TSH/PRL levels

Non-endocrine

Clear/green-brown

- Peri-areolar in location
- Gland of Montgomery
- +/− associated cystic mass
- Self-limited, resolves in 3–5 weeks with limited manipulation

Purulent

- Mastitis or abscess (see Breast abscess, Chapter 4, for management)

Fibrocystic

- Brown-green discharge
- Observation/symptomatic treatment

Bloody or serosanguinous nipple discharge

- Ductal ectasia
- Chronic cystic mastitis
- Fibrocystic changes
- Intraductal cysts
- Intraductal papillomas

    Definition: proliferation of cells in the mammary ducts that project into the ductal lumen

    Local trauma to vascular stalk may cause bloody discharge

    Ductogram to identify intraductal lesion – excise lesion

    Requires an experienced radiologist; can be quite painful

- Cystosarcoma phyllodes (rare)
- If bloody discharge with associated mass:

    Management:

    Excision vs fine-needle aspiration for persistent associated mass

35 Obesity

Evaluation of obesity in childhood:

> Offers the best hope for preventing disease progression with its associated morbidities

> While genetic and hormonal causes of obesity are rare, they do warrant consideration in obese children

> Obesity has a negative impact on the self-esteem of children and adolescents, with potential implications for long-term happiness and success in life.

> Directed sessions that emphasize healthy eating and exercise habits for children and their families may have lasting effects on the lifestyle of these patients

Definition

See Table 35-1

Differential diagnosis

Idiopathic vs endogenous obesity

Endogenous causes:

> Either hormonal or genetic defect

> Affects a very small percentage of children

> Can be inferred by a careful history and physical exam

> Characterized by growth failure; usually at or under the 5th percentile of height for age or significant drop off from the child's previous growth curve

> Hypothyroidism is the most frequent defect; diagnosed withelevated thyroid stimulating hormone (TSH) (and/or low freethyroxine level; associated constipation, cold intolerance, and dry skin

Table 35-1 Definitions of obesity and severe obesity

Index	Obesity	Severe obesity	Relevant information
Mean weight for height	> 120%	> 140%	Actual weight is 20% or more above the mean weight for children of this height
Weight for height	> 85 percentile	> 95 percentile	Readily available reference charts, easy to use but do not differentiate lean body mass from fat
Triceps skin fold	> 85 percentile	> 95 percentile	Direct measurement of subcutaneous fat, more accurate measurement of obesity but more intra-observer variability
Body mass index (kg/m^2)	85 percentile	95 percentile	Percentiles are age- and gender-specific, better correlates excess weight to fat in younger children and adolescents
Ponderal index (kg/m^3)	85 percentile	95 percentile	Percentiles are age- and gender-specific, better correlates excess weight to fat in older children

Used with permission from Moran R. Evaluation and treatment of childhood obesity. *Am Fam Physician* 1999;59:861–8. Adapted with permission from Williams CL, Campanaro LA, Squillace M, Bollella M. Management of childhood obesity in pediatric practice. *Ann N Y Acad Sci* 1997;817:225–40

Hypercortisolism (Cushing's syndrome); diagnosed with an elevated 24-hour urine free cortisol collection or dexamethasone suppression test:

- Give 1 mg of dexamethasone orally at bedtime and draw a plasma cortisol at 8 a.m.

A value of:

- < 6 µg/dl rules out Cushing's syndrome
- 6–10 µg/dl makes Cushing's syndrome unlikely
- > 10 µg/dl makes Cushing's syndrome diagnosis

Idiopathic causes:

Diagnosis of exclusion of above endogenous causes

EVALUATION

Office evaluation

Initial visit and yearly, measure height and weight and graph on age appropriate curve (see Figures 35-1, 35-2, 35-3, and 35-4)

At each visit check blood pressure with age appropriately sized blood pressure cuff (see Figure 35-5); if abnormal refer to primary care provider

Follow instructions in Figure 35-5

At each yearly visit: (if abnormal finding refer to appropriate specialist for further evaluation and management)

Evaluation for cardiac disease risk factors: family history of early (less than age 55) cardiovascular disease, high cholesterol, hypertension, and diabetes; cigarette smoking; level of physical activity

Evaluation for orthopedic issues: back or extremity problems

Evaluation for dermatologic problems: monilia, acanthosis nigricans, in axillary and perineal intertriginous areas

Evaluation for depression and other emotional issues

Evaluation for menstrual disorders

Laboratory tests

Lipid panel every two years in obese children (National Cholesterol Education Program Expert Panel on Blood Cholesterol Levels in Children and Adolescents). If abnormal consider nutritional consultation and rescreen in six months; if persistent refer to primary care provider

Consider screening at initial visit for hyperinsulinemia and glucose intolerance and as indicated in future visits; If abnormal refer to primary care provider or consult with pediatric endocrinology

INTERVENTION (MANAGEMENT)

See Tables 35-2 and 35-3

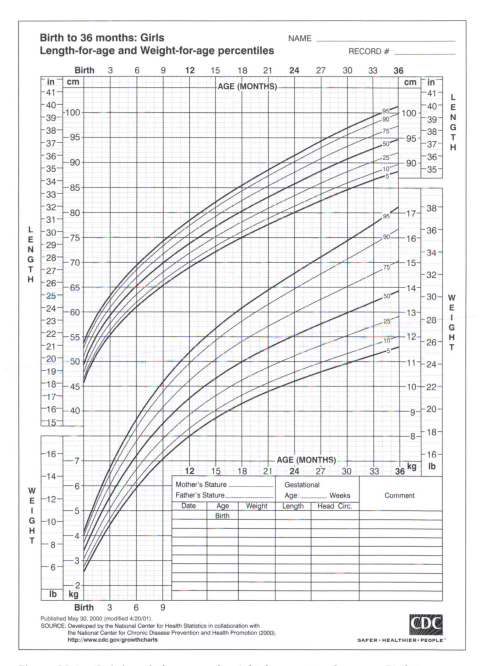

Figure 35-1   Girls length-for-age and weight-for-age growth curves. Birth to 36 months (5th–95th percentile). Used with permission from www.cdc.gov/nchs/ about/ nhanes/growthcharts/clinical/charts.htm

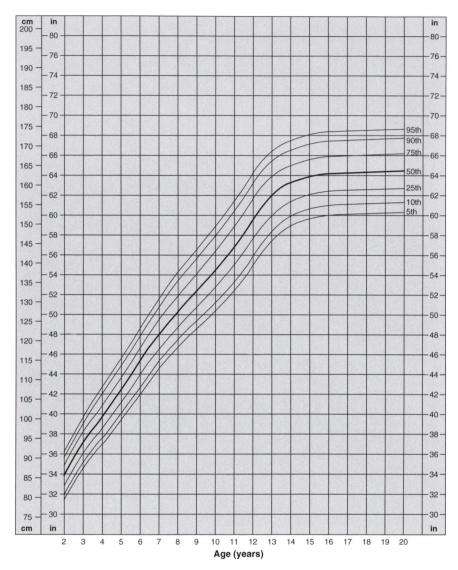

Figure 35-2   Girls stature-for-age and weight-for-age growth curves. 2 to 20 years (5th–95th percentile). Used with permission from www.cdc.gov/nchs/about/major/nhanes/growthcharts/clinical/charts.htm

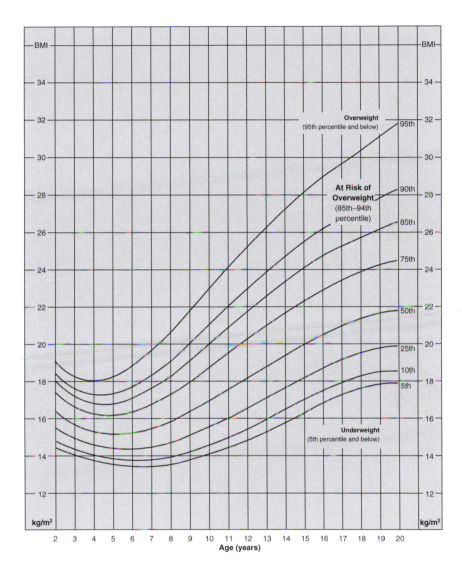

Figure 35-3 Body mass index for age. Used with permission from American College of Obstetricians and Gynecologists. *Tool Kit for Teen Care 2003*. Developed by the National Center for Health Statistics in Collaboration with the National Center for Chronic Disease Prevention and Health Promotion (2000)

Stature m (in)

Weight Kg (lb)	1.24 (49)	1.27 (50)	1.30 (51)	1.32 (52)	1.35 (53)	1.37 (54)	1.40 (55)	1.42 (56)	1.45 (57)	1.47 (58)	1.50 (59)	1.52 (60)	1.55 (61)	1.57 (62)	1.60 (63)	1.63 (64)	1.65 (65)	1.68 (66)	1.70 (67)	1.73 (68)	1.75 (69)	1.78 (70)	1.80 (71)	1.83 (72)	1.85 (73)	1.88 (74)	1.90 (75)	1.93 (76)
20 (45)	13	13	12	12	11	11	10	10	10	9	9	9	8															
23 (50)	15	14	13	13	12	12	12	11	11	10	10	10	9	9	9	9	9	8										
25 (55)	16	15	15	14	14	13	13	12	12	12	11	11	10	10	10	9	9	9										
27 (60)	18	17	16	16	15	15	14	13	13	13	12	12	11	11	11	10	10	10	9	9								
29 (65)	19	18	17	17	16	16	15	15	14	14	13	13	12	12	12	11	11	10	10	10	10							
32 (70)	21	20	19	18	17	17	16	16	15	15	14	14	13	13	12	12	12	11	11	11	10	10						
34 (75)	22	21	20	20	19	18	17	17	16	16	15	15	14	14	13	13	12	12	12	11	11	11	10					
36 (80)	24	22	21	21	20	19	19	18	17	17	16	16	15	15	14	14	13	13	13	12	12	11	11	11				
39 (85)	25	24	23	22	21	21	20	19	18	18	17	17	16	16	15	15	14	14	13	13	13	12	12	12	11			
41 (90)	27	25	24	23	22	22	21	20	19	19	18	18	17	17	16	16	15	15	14	14	13	13	13	12	12	12		
43 (95)	28	27	25	25	24	23	22	21	20	20	19	19	18	17	17	16	16	15	15	14	14	13	13	13	12	12		
45 (100)	29	28	27	26	25	24	23	22	22	21	20	20	19	18	18	17	17	16	16	15	15	14	14	14	13	13	13	12
48 (105)	31	30	28	27	26	25	24	24	23	22	21	21	20	19	19	18	17	17	16	16	16	15	15	14	14	13	13	13
50 (110)	32	31	30	29	27	27	25	25	24	23	22	22	21	20	19	19	18	18	17	17	16	16	15	15	15	14	14	13
52 (115)	34	32	31	30	29	28	27	26	25	24	23	23	22	21	20	20	19	18	18	17	17	16	16	15	15	14	14	
54 (120)	35	34	32	31	30	29	28	27	26	25	24	24	23	22	21	20	20	19	19	18	18	17	17	16	16	15	15	15
57 (125)	37	35	34	33	31	30	29	28	27	26	25	25	24	23	22	21	21	20	20	19	19	18	17	17	17	16	16	15
59 (130)	38	37	35	34	32	31	30	29	28	27	26	26	25	24	23	22	22	21	20	20	19	19	18	18	17	17	16	16
61 (135)	40	38	36	35	34	33	31	30	29	28	27	27	25	25	24	23	22	22	21	20	20	19	19	18	18	17	17	16
64 (140)	41	39	38	36	35	34	32	31	30	29	28	27	26	26	25	24	23	22	22	21	21	20	20	19	19	18	18	17
66 (145)	43	41	39	38	36	35	34	33	31	30	29	28	27	26	26	25	24	23	23	22	21	21	20	20	19	19	18	18
68 (150)	44	42	40	39	37	36	35	34	32	31	30	29	28	28	27	26	25	24	24	23	22	21	21	20	20	19	19	18
70 (155)	46	44	42	40	39	37	36	35	33	33	31	30	29	29	27	26	26	25	24	23	23	22	22	21	21	20	19	19
73 (160)	47	45	43	42	40	39	37	36	35	34	32	31	30	29	28	27	27	26	25	24	24	23	22	22	21	21	20	19
77 (170)	50	48	46	44	42	41	39	38	37	36	34	33	32	31	30	29	28	27	27	26	25	24	24	23	23	22	21	21
79 (175)	51	49	47	46	44	42	40	39	38	37	35	34	33	32	31	30	29	28	27	27	26	25	24	24	23	22	22	21
82 (180)		51	48	47	45	44	42	40	39	38	36	35	34	33	32	31	30	29	28	27	27	26	25	24	24	23	23	22
84 (185)			50	48	46	45	43	42	40	39	37	36	35	34	33	32	31	30	29	28	27	26	26	25	25	24	23	23
86 (190)			51	49	47	46	44	43	41	40	39	37	36	35	34	32	32	31	30	29	28	27	27	26	25	24	24	23
88 (195)				51	49	47	45	44	42	41	39	38	37	36	35	33	32	31	31	30	29	28	27	26	26	25	25	24
91 (200)					50	48	46	45	43	42	40	39	38	37	35	34	33	32	31	30	29	28	27	27	26	25	24	
93 (205)						50	47	46	44	43	41	40	39	38	36	35	34	33	32	31	30	29	29	28	27	26	26	25
95 (210)						51	49	47	45	44	42	41	40	39	37	36	35	34	33	32	31	30	29	28	28	27	26	26
98 (215)							50	48	46	45	43	42	41	40	38	37	36	35	34	33	32	31	30	29	28	28	27	26
100 (220)							51	49	47	46	44	43	42	40	39	38	37	35	35	33	33	31	31	30	29	28	28	27
102 (225)								51	49	47	45	44	42	41	40	38	37	36	35	34	33	32	31	30	30	29	28	27
104 (230)									50	48	46	45	43	42	41	39	38	38	36	36	34	34	33	32	31	30	29	28
107 (235)									51	49	47	46	44	43	42	40	39	38	37	36	35	34	33	32	31	30	30	29
109 (240)										50	48	47	45	44	43	41	40	39	38	36	36	34	34	33	32	31	30	29
111 (245)										51	49	48	46	45	43	42	41	39	38	37	36	35	34	33	32	31	31	30
113 (250)											50	49	47	46	44	43	42	40	39	38	37	36	35	34	33	32	31	30
116 (255)												50	48	47	45	44	42	41	40	39	38	37	36	35	34	33	32	31
118 (260)												51	49	48	46	44	43	42	41	39	39	37	36	35	34	33	33	32
120 (265)													50	49	47	45	44	43	42	40	39	38	37	36	35	34	33	32
122 (270)													51	50	48	46	45	43	42	41	40	39	38	37	36	35	34	33
125 (275)														51	49	47	46	44	43	42	41	39	38	37	36	35	35	33
127 (280)															50	48	47	45	44	42	41	40	39	38	37	36	35	34
129 (285)															50	49	47	46	45	43	42	41	40	39	38	37	36	35
132 (290)																50	48	47	46	44	43	42	41	39	38	37	36	35
134 (295)																50	49	47	46	45	44	42	41	40	39	38	37	36
136 (300)																	50	48	47	45	44	43	42	41	40	39	38	37

Reprinted with permission from: Guidelines for Adolescent Preventive Services (GAPS) Implementation Training Workbook. 2nd edition. Chicago, Illinois: American Medical Association, 1996

Figure 35-4 Body mass index chart. Used with permission from *Guidelines for Adolescent Preventative Services (GAPS).* © 1996, American Medical Association

Table 35-2 Preventing obesity: tips for parents

Respect your child's appetite: children do not need to finish every bottle or meal
Avoid pre-prepared and sugared foods when possible
Limit the amount of high-calorie foods kept in the home
Provide a healthy diet, with 30% or fewer calories derived from fat
Provide ample fiber in the child's diet
Skim milk may safely replace whole milk at 2 years of age
Do not provide food for comfort or as a reward
Do not offer sweets in exchange for a finished meal
Limit amount of television viewing
Encourage active play
Establish regular family activities such as walks, ball games and other outdoor activities

Used with permission from Moran R. Evaluation and treatment of childhood obesity.
Am Fam Physician 1999;59:861–8

Table 35-3 Components of a successful weight loss plan

Component	Comment
Reasonable weight-loss goal	Initially, 5 to 10 lb or a rate of 1 to 4 lb per month
Dietary management	Provide dietary prescription specifying total number of calories per day and recommended percentage of calories from fat, protein and carbohydrates
Physical activity	Begin according to child's fitness level, with ultimate goal of 20–30 minutes per day (in addition to any school activity)
Behavior modification	Self-monitoring, nutritional education, stimulus control, modification of eating habits, physical activity, attitude change, reinforcements and rewards
Family involvement	Review family activity and television viewing patterns, involve parents in nutrition counseling

Used with permission from Moran R. Evaluation and treatment of childhood obesity.
Am Fam Physician 1999;59:861–8

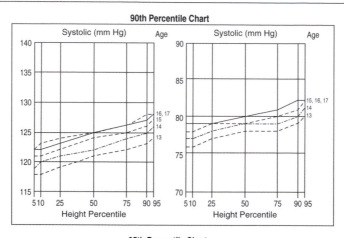

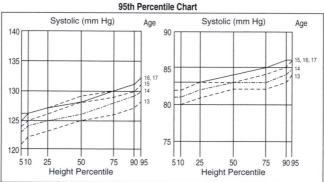

STEPS FOR ASSESSING CLASSIFICATION OF BLOOD PRESSURE

1. Use the standard height chart (on back) to determine the height percentile.
2. Measure the adolescent's blood pressure. Record systolic blood pressure (SBP) and diastolic blood pressure (DBP).
3. Find the adolescent's age on the right side of the 90th percentile chart for DBP. Follow the age line horizontally across the chart to the intersection of the line for the height percentile (vertical line).
4. Move up or down the height percentile line to the intersection of measured blood pressure.

Result on 90th Percentile Chart

- If you move down on the height percentile line, blood pressure is normal. Repeat steps 3 and 4 on the chart for 90th percentile SBP.
- If you move up on the height percentile line, you must repeat steps 3 and 4 on the chart for 95th percentile DBP.

(Continued)

Figure 35-5 Steps for assessing classification of blood pressure. Used with permission from American College of Obstetricians and Gynecologists. *Tool Kit for Teen Care 2003.* © ACOG

Figure 35-5 (*Continued*)

Result on 95th Percentile Chart

- If you move down on the height percentile line, blood pressure is high-normal. Repeat steps 3 and 4 on the chart for 95th percentile SBP.
- If you move up on the height percentile line, hypertension* is indicated. Repeat steps 3 and 4 on the chart for 95th percentile SBP.

*Note that hypertension is diagnosed after three consecutive blood pressure readings above the 95th percentile on three separate occasions.

Classification of Blood Pressure in Children and Adolescents*

SBP and DBP < 90th percentile	Normal
SBP and DBP ≥ 90th percentile and < 95th percentile	High-Normal†
SBP and DBP ≥ 95th percentile	Hypertension†

*For age and sex

†For age and sex measured on at least three separate occassions

SBP = systolic blood pressure

DBP = diastolic blood pressure

Modified from National High Blood Pressure Education Program. Update on the Task Force Report (1987) on High Blood Pressure in Children and Adolescents: a working group report from the National High Blood Pressure Education Program. National Institutes of Health, National Heart, Lung and Blood Institute. Bethesda, MD: National High Blood Pressure Education Program, 1996; NIH publication no. 96-3790.

BIBLIOGRAPHY

American College of Obstetricians and Gynecologists. *Tool Kit for Teen Care.* ACOG: Washington DC, 2003

Epstein LH, Myers MD, Raynor HA, *et al*. Treatment of pediatric obesity. *Pediatrics* 1998;101:554–70

Moran R. Evaluation and treatment of childhood obesity. *Am Fam Physician* 1999;59:861–8

36 Oncology patients and gynecologic issues

Reproductive function can be damaged partially or fully by the oncologic treatment modalities

Menstrual disorders, most commonly menorrhagia and amenorrhea, can result from the oncologic treatment modalities

Childhood cancer survivors have a 10% increased lifetime risk of a second malignancy; breast and ovarian cancer are among the most common

MANAGEMENT

Initial visit

(If possible prior to oncologic treatment)

Gynecologic, medical and family cardiovascular disease history

Physical exam: skin, thyroid, breasts and external genitalia (if not sexually active) or full pelvic (if sexually active); check with oncologist regarding pelvic exam if thrombocytopenia

Laboratory tests:

> Sexually active: pregnancy test, *Neisseria gonorrhoeae, Chlamydia trachomatis,* HIV, Hepatitis B (if not immunized) and rapid plasma reagin (RPR); pelvic ultrasound if bimanual limited

> Not sexually active: pelvic ultrasound if pelvis not imaged during oncologic work-up

Counseling and treatment

Reproductive function

Key points:

> Radiation can damage pelvic organs: ovarian failure; vaginal erosion and/or stenosis; vulvar erosion

> > • LD_{50} (median lethal dose) to oocyte is 400 rads

Chemotherapeutic agents can cause ovarian failure: predominantly alkylating agents but long, extended courses with other agents can also have an effect

- Particular agents: cyclophosphamide, chlorambucil, busulfan, melphalan, MOPP (mechlorethamine, vincristine, procarbazine, and prednisone), MVPP (nitrogen mustard, vinblastine, procarbazine, and prednisolone) and ChlVPP/EVA (chlorambucil, vinblastine, prednisolone, procarbazine, doxorubicin, and etoposide)

Counseling:

Use a multidisciplinary approach involving the medical oncologist, radiation oncologist, and gynecologist to best plan avoidance of complications and then present plan to patient and family

Contraception is important both during and after treatment in the sexually active patient, remembering that elevated liver function tests (LFTs), history of thromboembolic events are contraindications for the use of estrogen; thrombophilia work-up is necessary if there is a strong family history of early (< 55 years) cardiovascular disease (see Contraception, Chapter 11)

Counsel repeatedly regarding benefits of continuous abstinence while undergoing treatment; recognition of signs of early infection; what constitutes worrisome menstrual bleeding; need for condom use; and frequent gynecologic screening for sexually transmitted diseases in the sexually active patient

Treatment:

Radiation

- Oophoropexy: moving the ovaries out of the radiation field

  Should be planned with the radiation oncologist

  Even with good planning, radiation field can have some spread and damage gonadal tissue; small risk of compromise to ovarian blood supply with movement

  Do not move if there is a chance that tumor has invaded pelvic organs

  Post-therapy follicle stimulating hormone (FSH) level can be monitored to see if fertility is maintained; if FSH is consistently elevated, the diagnosis of premature ovarian failure is made; there are case reports where occasionally ovulation returns on a limited basis in future

  Would do laparoscopically unless staging laparotomy planned; use permanent suture

- Vagina and vulva can sometimes be protected from radiation-induced stenosis with use of topical estrogen cream in the postmenarcheal child
- Vulvar erosions can be treated with silvadene cream

Chemotherapy

- Small case series report the benefit of suppression of ovaries in a menstruating female with a gonadotropin releasing hormone (GnRH) agonist may prolong fertility after treatment

  Use 22.5 mg Lupron depot® IM every 3 months. If platelets less than 100 000/ml, hold pressure on site for 30 minutes to prevent hematoma formation with IM injections

  Expect significant withdrawal bleed 2–3 weeks after first injection

  Would add daily 5 mg norethindrone acetate if therapy prolonged over 6 months to protect bone loss

  Would check bone density pre-treatment and post-treatment if therapy prolonged (greater than 1 year)

  Would add daily 1500 mg calcium supplementation with onset of treatment to protect bone loss

Menstrual disorders

Key points:

  Menorrhagia can occur in menstruating adolescents when treatments cause significant anemia and/or thrombocytopenia and/or patient is anticoagulated

Counseling:

  Attempt to use multidisciplinary approach involving medical team (i.e. the medical oncologist, gynecologist, and primary care physicians), deciding how best to avoid these complications, and then present the management plan to the patient and family

Treatment:

  GnRH agonist: see above for treatment regimen

- Advantage: very effective after the first injection (often large withdrawal bleed 2–3 weeks after first injection); may see spotting occasionally with subsequent injection if counts are low)
- Disadvantages: IM injection can cause hematoma formation with decreased platelet count; bone loss; hot flashes and dizziness

  Oral contraceptive: cyclic or continuous fashion; use at least 30 µg preparation; avoid generics (may have increased breakthrough bleeding)

- Advantage: closest to normal cycling
- Disadvantages: may cause increase in LFTs or thromboembolic events; may not completely control bleeding (although never more than spotting)

Progestin only agents (Norethindrone minipills, Depo-Provera®, Megace®)

- Advantages: does not increase LFTs as easily as estrogens; does not effect thromboembolism
- Disadvantages: Minipill or Depo-Provera® may not control bleeding completely; Megace® (40 mg bid with increases every 2–3 days of 40 mg a day increments) will control bleeding but at high doses will significantly increase appetite and may result in obesity
- Depo-Provera® is an IM injection that can cause hematoma formation with decreased platelet count (hold pressure for 30 minutes if platelets less than 100 000/ml; prolonged use may effect bone loss (see Osteoporosis, Chapter 38) (consider bone density if treatment prolonged and causing amenorrhea for over a year; would recommend increased exercise and 1500 mg calcium intake). May need monthly injections initially to induce amenorrhea, and can take 6 months to one year to induce amenorrhea

Post-treatment counseling

Chemotherapy effects can last up to 1 year

May have amenorrhea after oncologic treatment

- Check for elevated FSH: ovarian failure; ongoing studies investigating the protective function of GnRH during treatment to prevent this
- If ovarian failure, check bone density; see Osteoporosis (Chapter 38)
- Occasionally ovaries will spontaneously ovulate after years of failure; use contraceptive not only for menstrual restoration but to protect from pregnancy when not desired

Emphasize importance of regular self-breast exam and gynecologic exams when age-appropriate

BIBLIOGRAPHY

Perlman SE, Emans SJ, Laufer MR. In Emans SJ, Laufer MR, Goldstein DP, eds. *Gynecologic Issues in Young Women With Chronic Diseases in Pediatric Adolescent Gynecology*, 4th edn. Philadelphia: Lippincott-Raven 1998:715–50

37 Operative care

Offer information

Separate office visit with parents and child to discuss the surgery

Tour of the operating room suite

Demonstrate procedure with anatomically correct dolls and other visual aids

Operative consent

Document in the medical record that you have discussed the reason for the procedure, the possible outcome if the procedure is not performed, alternatives to the procedure, the benefits and risks to the procedure

Discuss the potential for blood transfusion and issues of family donating blood

Bowel prep

Most cases only require npo status after midnight the night before surgery. Therefore, younger children should have surgery earlier in the day

If suspicious of diagnosis of cancer, if history of previous surgery or concern that significant bowel involvement (e.g. endometriosis of the bowel) consider bowel prep

Bowel prep (see Table 37-1 and Figure 37-1)

Laboratory tests

Pregnancy test in all menstruating girls

Complete blood count (CBC), type and screen in all patients for laparotomy

Table 37-1   Outpatient bowel prep

(1)   Drink a large glass (at least 8 ounces) of water or clear liquid each hour from 11 a.m. to 11 p.m. the day prior to the procedure
(2)   All meals should be clear liquids (starting with breakfast, if possible) and may include synthetic juices, carbonated beverages, weak coffee or tea with sugar, clear broths or bouillon, and clear gelatin dessert
(3)   Take one bottle of Citrate of Magnesia at noon
(4)   Take four Dulcolax tablets with at least 8 ounces of water or clear liquid at 4 p.m.
(5)   After midnight, nothing is to be taken by mouth until the procedure has been completed

NOTE: Should the citrate of Magnesia not be given around noon time, take it as soon as possible, followed in four hours by the Dulcolax tablets

Courtesy of University Pediatric Surgical Associates PSC, Louisville, KY

INTRAOPERATIVE CARE

Positioning

Unless vaginal instruments used, position supine even for laparoscopy

If use dorsal lithotomy prefer Allen stirrups (baby Allen for a child)

In/out cath or indwelling foley

Bair Hugger

OG tube can be considered

Examination under anesthesia

Dorsal lithotomy position either in Allen or candy cane stirrups. If use candy canes use size appropriate, do not position with greater than 90 degrees flexion of hips or knees

Examine other body parts as well: skin, thyroid gland, breast tissue, abdomen, record findings

Examine genitalia in systematic fashion and record findings carefully (see Gynecologic examination, pediatric patient, Chapter 21)

Have available:

- Dacron swabs, male urethral size to take all cultures
- Culture media for gonorrhea (chocolate agar), *Chlamydia trachomatis* (viral media), aerobic organisms, *Shigella*
- Kefzol 20 mg/kg IV as needed before vulvar biopsy and after cultures obtained

(1)   Admit to _____
       Age _____ Weight _____
(2)   Diet: Clear liquid as tolerated
(3)   Begin normal saline enemas/irrigations through functional ostomy until clear (circle
       age and volume)

AGE	VOLUME
Newborn	100 cc
1 year	150 cc
2 years	200 cc
3 years	250 cc
4 years	280 cc
6 years	350 cc
8 years	450 cc
10 years	500 cc
12 years	600 cc
14 years	700 cc
16 years	800 cc

Consult with M.D. re: irrigation of defunctionalized bowel

(4)   Golytley® 20 cc/kg PO/NG now X1————————cc
(5)   Give last 2 enemas/irrigations using 0.1% Kanamycin solution with volume as
       above according to patient age
(6)   Erythromycin base PO at 1300, 1400, 2300 (for 0800 surgery) (circle weight and
       dose)

WEIGHT	DOSE
0–7.5 kg	62.5 mg
7.6–15 kg	125 mg
15.1–30 kg	250 mg
> 30 kg	500 mg

(7)   Neomycin base PO at 1300, 1400, 2300 (for 0800) (circle weight and dose)

WEIGHT	DOSE
0–7.5 kg	62.5 mg
7.6–15 kg	125 mg
15.1–30 kg	250 mg
> 30 kg	500 mg

(8)   Preoperative antibiotics
>1 year:
Cefotetan® (30 mg/kg)————————mg IV on call to OR (maximum dose
2 grams)
≤ 1 year:
Ampicillin (25 mg/kg)————————mg IV on call to OR
AND
Gentamicin (2.5 mg/kg)————————mg IV on call to OR

Figure 37-1   Inpatient bowel prep. Adapted with permission from Kosair
Children's Hospital, Louisville, KY

- Vulvar biopsy: Keyes punch biopsy instruments (2–5 mm)
- Silver nitrate or needle point bovie for vulvar biopsy hemostasis
- Vaginoscopy equipment as below; take pictures as indicated

Rectoabdominal exam as indicated

- Anus will often lose tone when rectum full of stool under general anesthesia

Laparoscopy

Positioning:

- Children: supine position
- Adolescent: dorsal lithotomy position with Allen stirrups, in prolonged cases use sequential compression stockings

Prefer open laparoscopy technique

Consider pre-incision use of local anesthetic (e.g. lidocaine) to skin

In young infant do not instill more than two liters of CO_2 gas; in child do not allow the intra-abdominal pressure over 8–9 mmHg; in menstruating adolescent pressure limit should be 12–14 mmHg: ask anesthesia to advise of any respiratory difficulties; do not use nitrous oxide

Port placement

- In neonate or infant, place the central port above the umbilicus; ancillary ports 2 fingerbreadths above the umbilicus in the mid-clavicular line; prefer ≤ 5 mm ports
- In prepubertal children, place the central port above the umbilicus; ancillary ports 2 fingerbreadths below the umbilical ports in the mid-clavicular line; prefer ≤ 5 mm ports
- In adolescents, port placement as with the adult

Take pictures of normal and abnormal findings to keep in the medical record

Laparotomy

Use intermittent compression boots

Preoperative first generation cephalosporin prophylaxis (20 mg/kg/dose)

Prefer subcuticular 4-0 Vicryl skin closure if possible

Vaginoscopy

Use a 7.5–9.0 mm cystoscope 0° attached to a light source with sterile saline irrigation fluid as a distention media

Child in dorsal lithotomy position with slight Trendelenberg

With gentle pressure on the vulva around the endoscope the irrigating fluid will distend the intact vaginal canal with good demonstration of lacerations

POSTOPERATIVE CARE

Laparoscopy

For pain relief:

- Narcotic: Capital (Amarin Pharmaceuticals, Warren, NJ) 1 mg/kg/dose (dosing is by codeine), 12.5 mg/tsp; a brand of Tylenol with codeine but without the alcohol component, Tylenol (10–15 mg/kg/dose q 4–6 h) with codeine (0.5 mg/kg/dose q 4–6 h) or Tylenol with oxycodone (0.5–0.15 mg/kg/dose q 4 h)
- Non-narcotic: NSAIDs: motrin, ibuprofen, advil

    Child: 20–40 mg/kg/24 h in 3–4 divided doses

    Adolescent > 45 kg: 400–800 mg every 6–8 h

Incision(s) is typically closed with a subcuticular 4-0 Vicryl to avoid having to remove anything postoperatively

Avoid getting incision wet for 24 hours and any lifting over 5 lbs, and sexual activity until the postoperative visit 1–2 weeks later. This will vary with the age of patient and type of surgery

Laparotomy

If simple dissection, diet is clear liquids and advance as tolerated

Compression boots while in bed

For pain relief:

- If not contraindicated (i.e. renal insufficiency) one may consider Toradol (Roche Pharmaceuticals, Nutley, NJ) (adolescent > 45 kg load 30 mg, run at 15 mg every 6 h) intravenously for 48 h
- Should also use IV morphine prn

    Child: 0.1–0.2 mg/kg/dose every 2–4 h

    Adolescent > 45 kg: 2–15 mg every 2–6 h

- Once on po switch to oral NSAIDs and narcotics (as above)
- IV rates calculated: 40 ml (first 10 kg body weight) + 20 ml (second 10 kg body weight) + 10 ml (for every 10 kg body weight over that); a 45 kg adolescent should be able to follow adult fluid recommendations

  > For the very young infants use 5% dextrose and 0.2 NaCl and in older children use 5% dextrose and 0.45 NaCl

Incision is typically closed with a subcuticular 4-0 Vicryl to avoid having to remove anything postoperatively

Avoid getting incision wet for 24 hours and avoid lifting over 5 lbs, and sexual activity until the postoperative visit two weeks later. This will vary with the age of patient and type of surgery

Postoperative visit

Brief minimally invasive exam: abdomen, incision, extremities

Procedure is discussed in detail; utilize pictures taken

Discuss results of any tests, both positive and negative, including pathology

Be very reassuring and positive about the outcome with the patient and parents; children from approximately 18 months and older can have negative feelings and fears regarding their female organs that can have significant psychologic sequelae later in their life

38 Osteoporosis

Although defined by a z score of less than –2.00 on bone densitometry, there are very few studies or standards of measurement of bone density in children and adolescents

May be more useful to follow a trend between bone density scan results than a single value

Declining bone density needs aggressive treatment in the adolescent as this is time of peak bone mass accrual

Osteoporosis is associated with oncologic and renal disease; chronic steroid use; and idiopathic premature ovarian failure; possibly prolonged Depo-Provera® and Lupron Depot® use

DIAGNOSIS

History

> Menstrual history
>
> Medical history
>
> Medications
>
> Family gynecologic history
>
> Fracture history

Physical examination

> Measure height/weight/heart rate/blood pressure
>
> Evaluate for evidence of hypoestrogenism (atrophy) on external genitalia

Laboratory/imaging

> Luteinizing hormone (LH), follicle stimulating hormone (FSH), estradiol to assess for ovarian failure as well
>
> Bone densitometry

MANAGEMENT

Consult with pediatric endocrinology

Consider oral contraceptive use (any dose, monophasic preferred)

Actonel (dosing should be prescribed in conjunction with a pediatric endocrinologist) is given once a day at least 30 minutes before food or drink except water. The patient should be instructed to swallow while upright with 6–8 oz (180–240 ml) of water and to not lie down for 30 minutes. Use is cautioned in patients with renal disease

Supplement calcium (1300–1600 mg per day)

Vitamin D (400–800 IU qd)

Exercise (weight bearing): 20–30 minutes per day at least 5 days per week

Monitoring

Can follow effectiveness with 6 month urine N-telopeptide measurement

Use first bone density measurement as the patient's baseline for further tests; do not repeat more frequently than every 12–18 months

Prevention

Early identification of risk factors (in order of importance): disease states, medication, poor nutrition, family history, and menstrual dysfunction

Closely monitor menstrual cycle, level of strenuous activity if irregular menses noted, height/weight growth patterns

Counsel:

- Participate in moderate physical activity and exercise
- Eat a well-balanced diet that meets the recommended daily allowance for calcium and vitamin D; avoid disordered eating patterns
- Limit alcohol intake
- Encourage tobacco cessation

BIBLIOGRAPHY

Gordon CM. Bone density issues in the adolescent gynecology patient. *J Pediatr Adolesc Gynecol* 2000;13:157–61

39 Ovarian/adnexal torsion

DEFINITION

Rotation of the ovary or adnexa around the vascular pedicle resulting in obstruction of the arterial, venous, and lymphatic flow to ovary and eventual ovarian/tubal infarction if undiagnosed and treated

KEY POINTS

Ovarian/adnexal torsion is a surgical emergency due to the potential for reproductive/hormonal compromise

Prompt diagnosis is important to establish diagnosis and provide intervention to salvage the involved structures from infarction

Signs and symptoms are variable and non-specific

Need to have high index of suspicion in this age group

Under age 5, 25% of all ovarian torsion cases are spontaneous with no ovarian pathology and have a predominance on the right side

Most cases of torsion involve an underlying cystic or solid mass although it may occur without definitive etiology

Ovarian masses with torsion are typically benign

Most malignancies present with an abdominal mass **not** torsion

COMMON PRESENTATION

Complex mass with acute abdominal pain often closely followed with onset of nausea and vomiting, eventual low-grade fever and mildly elevated white blood cell count

Presentation easily confused with acute appendicitis or other intraperitoneal processes, thereby creating a delay in diagnosis

Malignant tumors unlikely to present with torsion

DIFFERENTIAL DIAGNOSIS

Appendicitis – nausea/vomiting several hours after pain

Gastroenteritis – may see associated diarrhea; other family members with similar symptoms

Ectopic pregnancy

Pelvic inflammatory disease – symptoms more gradual

Hemorrhagic ovarian cysts

Renal stone – more costovertebral angle tenderness; urine with large blood

DIAGNOSIS

History

Characterize pain:

- Location
- Quality
- Duration (can wax/wane)

Nausea/vomiting/anorexia (common)

Past medical history:

- Previous torsion
- Abdominal surgery
- Inflammatory bowel disease

Confidential sexual history

Physical examination

Vital signs:

Look for fever/tachycardia

Abdomen:

Tenderness/mass/hernia

Pelvic:

Uterine/adnexal enlargement/tenderness

Sexually transmitted disease evaluation as indicated

Imaging

Ultrasound:

- Typically the affected ovary is enlarged with multiple small follicles along its periphery reflecting the congestion of the involved ovary and transudation of fluid into follicles due to circulatory impairment
- This finding has 64% sensitivity and 97% specificity
- Other findings may be a complex mass with septation and debris or cystic mass
- IF solid mass found as part of torsed adnexa:

    Draw tumor markers (see Ovarian masses and tumors, Chapter 41) to assist in planning management (detorsion with cystectomy vs salpingo-oophorectomy (S&O))

    IF positive tumor markers – consider S&O

Doppler flow study:

- Can show decreased or no venous or arterial flow. Normal flow to ovary does not necessarily exclude the diagnosis

MANAGEMENT

If torsion suspected:

- Prompt surgical evaluation/management indicated
- Either open laparotomy or laparoscopic approach:

    Untwist and conserve tubo-ovarian tissue:
    (Even those ovaries that look blue-black/necrotic in appearance)

    Appropriately counsel parents about rare possibility of hidden malignancy within ovary and possibility of postoperative fever and rare possibility of repeat surgery

    Ovarian bivalving after detorsion has been described as a possible technique to decrease ovarian intracapsular pressure, allow for increased arterial perfusion and thereby facilitating adnexal reperfusion and recovery

    Oophoropexy with permanent suture:

    No evidence that decreases incidence of recurrence or contralateral torsion/no literature to state that it causes harm

    Theoretically could cause adhesions/distortion of ovary–tube relationship

May consider use in recurrent cases or in cases in which no etiology can be determined

Post-operative course:

If adnexa is untwisted:

Patient likely to have slow recovery over 48–72 h accompanied by fevers and increased white blood cell count that decreases over that time while the ovarian damage/tissue necrosis is corrected at the cellular level

Should the patient worsen/not improve over 72 h – repeat surgery with possible excision of affected adnexal structure would be indicated

Recommend follow-up ultrasound at 4–6 weeks and 4–6 months

BIBLIOGRAPHY

Cass DL, Hawkins E, Brandt ML, *et al.* Surgery for ovarian masses in infants, children and adolescents: 102 consecutive patients treated in a 15 year period. *J Pediatr Surg* 2001;36:693–9

Cohen Z, Shinhar D, Kopernik G, *et al.* The laparoscopic approach to uterine adnexal torsion in childhood. *J Pediatr Surg* 1996;31:1557–9

Dolgin SE. Letter to the editor: Acute ovarian torsion in children. *Am J Surg* 2002;183:95–100

Dolgin SE, Lublin M, Shlasko E. Maximizing ovarian salvage when treating idiopathic adnexal torsion. *J Pediatr Surg* 2000;35:624–6

Goldstein DP. Ovarian neoplasms in infants, children and adolescents. In Rose BD, ed. *UpToDate*, Wellesley, MA: Up To Date, 2002

Hurh PJ, Meyer JS, Shaaban A. Ultrasound of a torsed ovary: characteristic gray-scale appearance despite normal and venous flows on Doppler. *Pediatr Radiol* 2002;32:586–8

Kokosha ER, Keller MS, Weber TR. Acute ovarian torsion in children. *Am J Surg* 2000;180:462–5

Kurzbart E, Mares AJ, Cohen Z, *et al.* Isolated torsion of the fallopian tube in premenarcheal girls. *J Pediatr Surg* 1994;29:1384–5

Styer AK, Laufer MR. Ovarian bivalving after detorsion. *Fertil Steril* 2002;77:1053–5

Templeman C, Hertweck SP, Fallat ME. The clinical course of unresected ovarian torsion. *J Pediatr Surg* 1993;35:1385–7

40 Ovarian cysts

Ovarian cysts are a consequence of normal follicular growth and development and when detected by ultrasound have a low incidence of complications including malignancy

Ovarian cysts are common in premenarcheal and adolescent girls

Usually 2–3 mm in size but can reach 17 mm diameter, rare > 20 mm

The majority of both simple and complex cysts resolve in 6 months without treatment

Modern management of ovarian cysts in neonates, prepubescent and adolescent girls is based on conservative treatment and close observation

FETAL OVARIAN CYSTS

Obstetrical ultrasound allows opportunity to diagnose *in utero* ovarian cysts that would have otherwise gone undetected

Differential diagnosis of cystic masses in female fetus/newborn

Ovarian cyst

Gastrointestinal etiology

- Intestinal duplication

- Intestinal obstruction

- Cystic meconium peritonitis

- Omental cyst

- Mesenteric cyst

- Choledochal cyst

Gynecologic

- Hydrometrocolpos

Urologic

- Urachal cyst
- Hydronephrosis
- Renal cyst
- Bladder distention

Complications

Rare and include: cyst enlargement with visceral compression, polyhydramnios, cyst rupture with hemorrhage, ovarian loss from torsion or autoamputation

Management

Observation:

High-resolution rate in neonatal period

Low risk of antenatal complications

Antenatal aspiration: **not** indicated

Defer treatment until neonatal period

Allow vaginal delivery:

No support to indicate operative delivery

NEONATAL OVARIAN CYSTS

Usually unilateral

Can be simple/complex

Complex cyst characterized by: cystic with fluid-debris level

cystic with retracting clot

septated with/without internal echoes

an echogenic wall

Complex ovarian cysts – usually represent *in utero*/neonatal torsion or hemorrhage

Differential diagnosis same as for fetuses (see above)

Both simple and complex cysts well documented to undergo regression within First 4 months of life

Malignancy is rare under the age of 2 years

Complications

Mass effect at diaphragm causing respiratory distress

Urinary tract or gastrointestinal obstruction

Ovarian torsion and necrosis

Intracystic hemorrhage

Incarceration in inguinal hernia

Management

Serial ultrasounds every 4–6 weeks

Educate caregivers re: signs of torsion:	Acute abdominal pain
	Nausea/vomiting
	Fever

Failure to regress: Possible non-ovarian cause

                Possible ovarian torsion, rare malignancy

Percutaneous aspiration:	Prophylactic for large cysts > 5 cm
Surgical indications:	Complex masses without involution over 4–6 months
	Recurrent cysts after aspiration
	Acute abdominal symptoms
Surgical technique:	Cystectomy
	Maximize ovarian salvage
	Laparoscopy safe/advantageous
	Harmonic scalpel works well for incision of ovarian capsule, traction counter-traction technique with use of suction irrigator

(See Figure 40-1)

CHILDHOOD OVARIAN CYSTS

35% incidence simple cysts in girls age 2–9 years

Microcysts (< 9 mm) resolve over 6 months

10% of cysts > 9 mm persist beyond 6 months

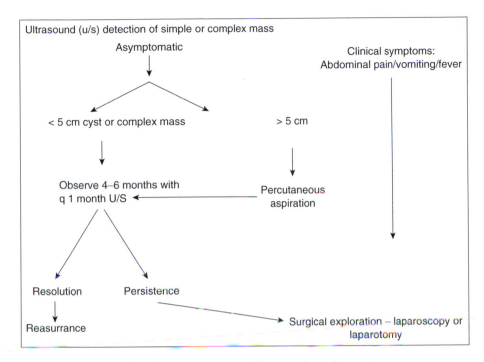

Figure 40-1 Algorithm for management of neonatal ovarian cysts

Can be associated with precocious puberty

Evaluate patient for breast development/vaginal bleeding

Can be secondary to an autonomously functioning ovarian cyst (e.g. McCune-Albright syndrome or hypothyroidism) or gonadotropin induced (see Precocious puberty, Chapter 51)

Most simple and complex masses in this age group resolve, even when > 5 cm

Solid/complex masses/masses without regression:

Most frequently are mature cystic teratomas

Malignancy possible in approximately 10% cases; germ cell tumors most common

(See Ovarian masses and tumors, Chapter 41)

Presentation

Asymptomatic mass

Incidental finding on ultrasound

Increasing abdominal girth

Acute abdominal pain with nausea, vomiting, fever (torsion)

Evaluation

Ultrasound

    If suspect torsion: Doppler flow

- Absent or decreased flow is suspicious for torsion
- (See Ovarian torsion, Chapter 39)

Management

Based on size, symptoms and composition seen on ultrasound:

Small, simple cysts (< 2 cm):	Normal findings
	Require no intervention
More than one small cyst:	Look for breast development
	Could be associated with isolated premature thelarche

Larger mass purely cystic/few internal echoes suggestive of hemorrhage without complex features (septation/calcification): Monitor q 4–8 weeks by ultrasound

                                                              Regression likely

Surgical indications:	Acute symptoms
	Solid or complex masses (See Ovarian masses and tumors, Chapter 41)
	Masses (> 2 cm) that fail to undergo regression over several months

ADOLESCENT OVARIAN CYSTS

Presentation

Asymptomatic

Menstrual irregularities

Pelvic pain

Urinary frequency

Constipation

Pelvic heaviness

With rupture/bleeding:

    Abdominal pain

With torsion:

Acute pain with nausea/vomiting/fever/leukocytosis

(See Ovarian torsion, Chapter 39)

Differential diagnosis

Ovarian cysts:

Follicular cysts

Corpus luteum cysts

Hemorrhagic functional cysts

Endometriomas

Benign/malignant neoplasms

Pathology mimicking ovarian cysts:

Disorders of the fallopian tube:

- Hydrosalpinx
- Pyosalpinx
- Paratubal cyst
- Ectopic pregnancy
- Tubal torsion

Obstructive genital lesions:

- Imperforate hymen
- Blind uterine horn
- Mullerian remnants

Peritoneal cysts

Periappendiceal abscesses

Evaluation

History

Weight gain/loss, vague abdominal pain – may suggest neoplastic process

Menstrual history – dysmenorrhea (pain with menses) may signal endometriosis or congenital obstructive anomalies

Confidential sexual history – may suggest an infectious process (i.e. tuboovarian abscess (TOA))

Physical examination

Include pelvic exam

Rule out pregnancy, sexually transmitted diseases (STDs)

Laboratory tests

Human chorionic gonadotropin (hCG), complete blood count (CBC), STD testing

Imaging

Ultrasound:	Presence of calcification suggests a teratoma
CT Scanning:	Can clarify images/helpful to distinguish gastrointestinal disorders (e.g. appendicitis) from ovarian
MRI:	Can delineate complicated uterine anomalies

Management

Based on:	Low rate of malignancy
	High incidence functional cysts/benign germ cell tumors
	Size: < 8 cm less likely for torsion, would observe
	> 8 cm, would advocate surgical intervention
Simple/complex adnexal masses	Observe for 2 to 3 menstrual cycles
Corpus luteal cysts	Repeat ultrasound
	Functional/hemorrhagic cysts resolve
	Oral contraceptives not helpful in resolution of current cyst but may prevent new onset cysts
Persistent/increasing/ symptomatic cysts	Surgical intervention for diagnosis/treatment
	Laparoscopic approach offers decreased surgical morbidity, outpatient management, and rapid recovery
	Aspiration associated with recurrence
	Recommend cystectomy with ovarian preservation even in cases of mature cystic teratomas

Ovarian masses with findings suspicious for malignancy:

- Multiloculated masses with papillations

- Solid components

- Increased blood flow

Manage as per ovarian masses (see Ovarian masses and tumors, Chapter 39)

If ovarian cyst with acute abdominal pain/fever/nausea – suspect torsion:

Evaluate surgically

BIBLIOGRAPHY

Cohen HL, Eisenberg P, Mandel F, *et al*. Ovarian cysts are common in premenarchal girls: A sonographic study of 101 children 2–12 years old. *Am J Roentgenol* 1992:159:89–91

Freedman SM, Kreitzer PM, Elkowitz SS, *et al*. Ovarian microcysts in girls with isolated premature thelarche. *J Pediatr* 1993;122:246–9

Goldstein DP. Ovarian neoplasms in infants, children and adolescents. In Rose BD, ed. Wellesley, MA: Up To Date, 2002

Millar DM, Blake JM, Stringer DA, *et al*. Prepubertal ovarian cyst formation: 5 years' experience. *Obstet Gynecol* 1993;81:434–8

Nussbaum AR, Sanders RC, Hartman DS, *et al*. Neonatal ovarian cysts: sonographic–pathologic correlation. *Radiology* 1988;158:817–21

Strickland JL. Ovarian cysts in neonates, children and adolescents. *Curr Opin Obstet Gynecol* 2002;14:459–65

Templeman CL, Hertweck SP, Scheetz JP, *et al*. The management of mature cystic teratomas in children and adolescents: a retrospective analysis. *Hum Reprod* 2000;15:2669–72

Warner BW, Kuhn JC, Barr LL. Conservative management of large ovarian cysts in children: The value of serial pelvic ultrasonography. *Surgery* 1992;112: 749–55

41 Ovarian masses and tumors

Solid ovarian masses are uncommon in childhood

Risk of malignancy increases with solid tumors

- Patients with malignancy usually present with asymptomatic mass
- May present with endocrine disturbance
- Advanced malignancies in children and teens are uncommon

Two-thirds of solid masses are germ cell tumors (the most common solid tumors)

- Most germ cell tumors are benign mature teratomas (dermoids)
- Dysgerminoma is the most common malignant germ cell tumor

Remaining one-third are sex cord tumors or epithelial tumors

- Sex cord tumors are usually hormonally active, presenting with precocious puberty, masculinization or dysfunctional bleeding

In cases of malignancy the goal of surgery is:

- Thorough removal of tumor and proper staging
- Sparing the normal ovary and tube if unaffected
- Biopsy of suspicious areas

DIFFERENTIAL DIAGNOSIS

Ovarian tumor

- Germ cell tumors

    Mature teratoma (dermoid)

    Immature teratoma

Dysgerminoma

Endodermal sinus tumor

Embryonal carcinoma

Choriocarcinoma

- Sex cord/stromal tumors

    Granulosa-thecal cell tumors

    Sertoli-stromal tumors

- Epithelial tumors

Neuroblastoma

Wilms' tumor

Rhabdomyosarcoma

Lymphoma

Leukemia

Endometrioma

DIAGNOSIS

Presentation

Most commonly abdominal pain or mass

Increasing abdominal girth

Nausea/vomiting

Precocious puberty

Masculinization

Dysfunctional uterine bleeding

Asymptomatic mass found on examination

Non-specific symptoms

History

Characterization of pain

- If acute and associated with symptoms of nausea/vomiting/fever may indicate torsion

Gastrointestinal/urologic symptoms

Onset of pubertal development

- Precocious (< age 8 years)

Menstrual/sexual history

Family history: Endometriosis

                     Inflammatory bowel disease

                     Ovarian tumors

Prior abdominal/pelvic surgery

Prior pelvic infections

Physical examination

Vital signs

General/pubertal development

Abdominal exam: Assess for areas of tenderness/signs of peritonitis

                     Characterize mass

Pelvic exam: External genitalia (assess pubertal development: whether age appropriate)

                     In child/anxious adolescent – rectoabdominal exam

                     In adolescent – rectovaginal-abdominal exam

Imaging

Ultrasound: Determine size of mass

                     Simple/complex/solid/bilateral

                     Identify calcifications

                     Any association with fluid

                     Doppler may determine pattern of blood flow

CT/MRI: Further delineation of mass/liver/lymphatic involvement

                     Helps define full extent of disease

Additional testing

Tumor markers: Many tumors in this age group will secrete protein markers

Draw:	Produced by:
Alpha-fetoprotein (AFP):	Endodermal sinus tumors
	Mixed germ cell tumors
	Immature teratomas
(*Note*: AFP can be increased until 8 months of age)	
Lactate dehydrogenase (LDH)	Dysgerminomas
Human chorionic gonadatropin	Dysgerminomas
	Hydatidiform moles
	Placental site tumors
	Choriocarcinomas
	Embryonal ovarian carcinoma
Carcinoembryonic antigen (CEA)	Germ cell tumors
	Epithelial ovarian carcinoma
Inhibin	Granulosa cell tumors
Mullerian inhibiting substance (MIS)	Granulosa cell tumors
CA–125/CA-19	Nonspecific marker for epithelial ovarian carcinoma

MANAGEMENT

Treatment

Surgical intervention:

- IF solid lesion with no available tumor markers and no evidence of malignancy intraoperatively (extracapsular extension, lymph node, omental involvement):

  Perform cystectomy with subsequent salpingo-oophorectomy if tumor markers return elevated or final path malignant

- IF suspect dermoid (shadowing echodensity/regional bright echoes on ultrasound):

  Laparoscopy/laparotomy for ovarian cystectomy

- IF tumor markers negative and at time of surgery ovarian appearance suspicious but unable to get frozen section to confirm malignancy:

  Consult with parents about possible need for second surgical procedure if final path malignant

  Do unilateral salpingo-oophorectomy with second staging procedure if final pathology returns malignant

- IF tumor markers positive, CT/MRI indicative of malignancy:

  Consult preoperatively with pediatric surgery and/or oncology

  Use sequential compression stockings

  Use vertical incision to allow surgical staging

  Preserve reproductive/sexual function as much as possible

  Perform adequate staging with unilateral salpingo-oophorectomy:

  > Examine ascites for malignant cells
  >
  > Inspect peritoneal/solid organ surfaces/biopsy suspicious areas
  >
  > Remove omentum
  >
  > Sample periaortic/pelvic lymph nodes
  >
  > Biopsy other ovary if suspicious

Management principles

Treat all malignancies in conjunction with gynecologic or pediatric oncology

- Germ cell tumors:

Teratoma (dermoid):	Most common germ cell tumor
	Usually benign – respond to cystectomy
	1% are immature and malignant
	Survival inversely related to grade
	Stage I Grade I – 90% survival
	Stage I Grade III – 30% survival
	Surgery alone for low grade–stage disease
	Chemotherapy for higher grade
Dysgerminoma:	If confined to ovary (Stage I) – 95% cure rate

	Other stages – 75% cure rate
	Bilateral 10–15% cases
	Unilateral salpingo-oophorectomy and careful exam of contralateral ovary
	Adjuvant chemotherapy:
	Bleomycin–etoposide–platinol
	Preserves fertility
Endodermal sinus tumor:	Also called yolk-sac tumor
	Most aggressive germ cell tumor
	Rapid spread to lymphatics
	Propensity for liver/lung/central nervous system metastases
	15% survival rate
	Unilateral salpingo-oophorectomy with staging as above
	With advanced disease – cytoreductive surgery indicated
	Adjuvant chemotherapy for all stages:
	Bleomycin–etoposide–platinol
Embryonal carcinoma:	Stage I – 50% survival rate
	Treat as with endodermal sinus tumor
Choriocarcinoma:	Rare to present in a child
	Usually presents during a pregnancy
	Treatment with excision/staging as above
	hCG is good marker for response to treatment
	Chemotherapy:
	Bleomycin–etoposide–platinol *or*
	Methotrexate–dactinomycin–cyclophosphamide

- Non-germ cell malignancies:

| Juvenile granulosa-thecal cell tumor: | Malignancy related to amount of granulosa cells present |

	Usually present with precocious puberty/menorrhagia
	Stage I – treat with surgery alone; survival nearly 100%
	> Stage I – multimodal therapy; survival 80%
Sertoli-Leydig cell tumors:	Rare
	Usually present with androgen excess (hirsutism, acne, amenorrhea, virilization)
	Testosterone is a good marker
	Vary in malignant potential
Epithelial tumors:	Uncommon in this age group
	Frequently bilateral
	Limited surgery may not be possible
	Adjuvant chemotherapy recommended with advanced disease

BIBLIOGRAPHY

Brown MF, Hebra A, McGeehin K, *et al*. Ovarian masses in children: a review of 91 cases of malignant and benign masses. *J Pediatr Surg* 1993;28:930–2

Cass DL, Hawkins E, Brandt ML, *et al*. Surgery for ovarian masses in infants, children and adolescents: 102 consecutive patients treated in a 15-year period. *J Pediatr Surg* 2001;36:693–9

Goldstein DP. Ovarian neoplasms in infants, children, and adolescents. In Rose BD, ed. *UpToDate*, Wellesley, MA: Up To Date, 2002

Lazar EL, Stolar CJH. Evaluation and management of pediatric solid ovarian tumors. *Semin Pediatr Surg* 1998;7:29–34

Patel MD, Feldstein VA, Lipson SD, *et al*. Cystic teratomas of the ovary: Diagnostic value of sonography. *Am J Roentgenol* 1998;171:1061–5

42 Pap testing

Non-sexually active adolescents:

> Screening to begin no later than age 21 (American Cancer Society Detection Guidelines 2002)

Sexually active adolescents:

> Screen approximately 3 years after onset of vaginal intercourse (American Cancer Society Detection Guidelines 2002)

> Yearly Pap testing in all sexually active teens especially the following:
> - Adolescents with early sexual debut/multiple partners
> - Immunosuppressed adolescents either by disease or medication
> - Adolescents with a history of sexual abuse with penetration

After initial Pap testing:

> Testing should occur every year thereafter if regular Pap tests are used or every 2 years thereafter if liquid-based cytology is used (American Cancer Society Detection Guidelines 2002); many adolescent providers prefer to repeat yearly despite the method

When Pap testing results dictate colposcopic evaluation, in addition to cervical evaluation, the vulva and vagina should also be examined for lesions requiring biopsy

Encourage smoking cessation due to relationship between smoking, human papillomavirus (HPV) acquisition, and abnormal Pap test results (see Substance abuse, Chapter 57)

Consider HIV testing on a yearly basis in patients with cervical intraepithelial neoplasia (CIN) 2–3

2001 BETHESDA SYSTEM

(see NCI web site at www.nci.nih.gov/newscenter/bethesda2001)

Table 42-1 Definitions of terms utilized in the consensus guidelines

Colposcopy is the examination of the cervix, vagina, and, in some instances the vulva, with the colposcope after the application of a 3–5% acetic acid solution coupled with obtaining colposcopically-directed biopsies of all lesions suspected of representing neoplasia.

Endocervical sampling includes obtaining a specimen for either histological evaluation using an endocervical curette or a cytobrush or for cytological evaluation using a cytobrush.

Endocervical assessment is the process of evaluating the endocervical canal for the presence of neoplasia using either a colposcope or endocervical sampling.

Diagnostic excisional procedure is the process of obtaining a specimen from the transformation zone and endocervical canal for histological evaluation and includes laser conization, cold-knife conization, loop electrosurgical excision (i. e., LEEP), and loop electrosurgical conization.

Satisfactory colposcopy indicates that the entire squamocolumnar junction and the margin of any visible lesion can be visualized with the colposcope.

Endometrial sampling includes obtaining a specimen for histological evaluation using an endometrial biopsy or a "dilatation and curettage" or hysteroscopy.

The Consensus Guidelines algorithms originally appeared in and are reprinted from *The Journal of Lower Genital Tract Disease*, Volume 16, issue 2, and are reprinted with the permission of ASCCP. © American Society for Colposcopy and Cervical Pathology 2002. No copies of the algorithms may be made without the prior consent of ASCCP

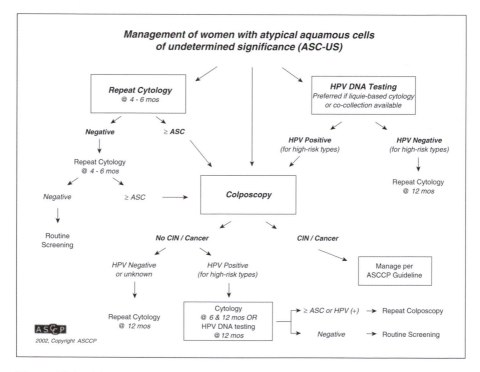

Figure 42-1 Management of women with atypical squamous cells of undetermined significance (ASC-US). The Consensus Guidelines algorithms originally appeared in and are reprinted from *The Journal of Lower Genital Tract Disease*, Volume 16, issue 2, and are reprinted with the permission of ASCCP. © American Society for Colposcopy and Cervical Pathology 2002. No copies of the algorithms may be made without the prior consent of ASCCP

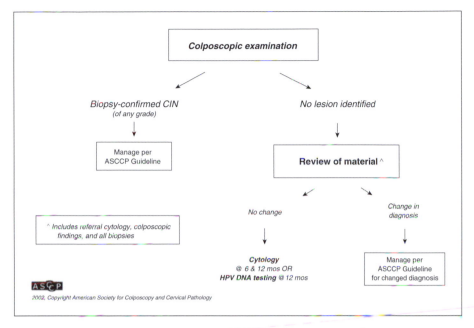

Figure 42-2   Management of women with atypical squamous cells: cannot exclude high-grade SIL (ASC-H). The Consensus Guidelines algorithms originally appeared in and are reprinted from *The Journal of Lower Genital Tract Disease*, Volume 16, issue 2, and are reprinted with the permission of ASCCP. © American Society for Colposcopy and Cervical Pathology 2002. No copies of the algorithms may be made without the prior consent of ASCCP

Management of cytologic abnormalities

See Table 42-1 for definitions of terms and for ASCCP algorithms see Figures 42-1, 42-2, 42-3, 42-4, 42-5, and 42-6

Management of cervical histologic abnormalities

See Table 42-2

CIN 1

Routine use of diagnostic excisional/ablative procedures is unacceptable for the initial management of patients with LSIL in the absence of biopsy-confirmed CIN

Biopsy confirmed CIN 1 (negative endocervical curettage (ECC))

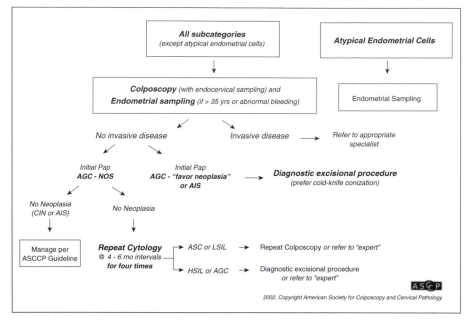

Figure 42-3 Management of women with atypical glandular cells (AGC). The Consensus Guidelines algorithms originally appeared in and are reprinted from *The Journal of Lower Genital Tract Disease*, Volume 16, issue 2, and are reprinted with the permission of ASCCP. © American Society for Colposcopy and Cervical Pathology 2002. No copies of the algorithms may be made without the prior consent of ASCCP

- Repeat regular Pap test every six months *or*
- Repeat liquid based Pap test with HPV typing yearly *or*
- HPV typing yearly

If still LSIL on Pap testing, repeat colposcopy

- Literature is limited on how long one can follow an adolescent with persistence before excisional/ablative procedure should be performed, some authors recommend one or two years
- Follow up after excisional/ablative procedure performed; literature is also very limited on recommended follow-up
- If negative cytology times two or negative HPV typing, return to yearly regular Pap testing or every two years liquid based Pap testing

CIN 2,3

Biopsy confirmed CIN 2*,3 (negative ECC):

- Loop electrosurgical excision (LEEP)/cryotherapy** (see below for procedures)

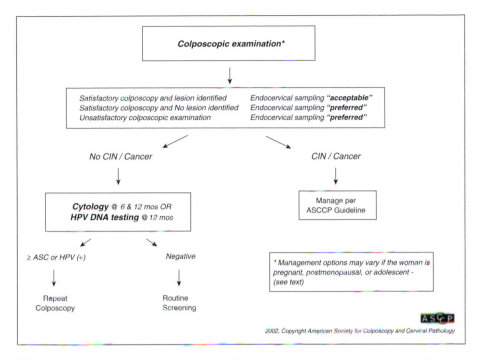

Figure 42-4 Management of women with low-grade squamous intraepithelial lesions (LSIL). The Consensus Guidelines algorithms originally appeared in and are reprinted from *The Journal of Lower Genital Tract Disease*, Volume 16, issue 2, and are reprinted with the permission of ASCCP. © American Society for Colposcopy and Cervical Pathology 2002. No copies of the algorithms may be made without the prior consent of ASCCP

5 mm depth CIN 2

8–10 mm CIN 3

*The 2001 Consensus Guidelines Conference state that observation is appropriate for properly counseled adolescents with biopsy-confirmed CIN 2 considered to be reliable for follow-up

**Some authors prefer the excisional procedure to rule out any microinvasive disease especially if lesion is large

Biopsy confirmed CIN 2,3 (positive ECC):

- Confirm with pathologist positive ECC not contaminant from cervical biopsy
- Confirmed ECC positive

    Lesion completely visualized: LEEP

    Lesion not completely visualized: cold knife cone biopsy

Biospy confirmed CIS (squamous cell carcinoma or adenocarcinoma)

- Cold knife cone biopsy

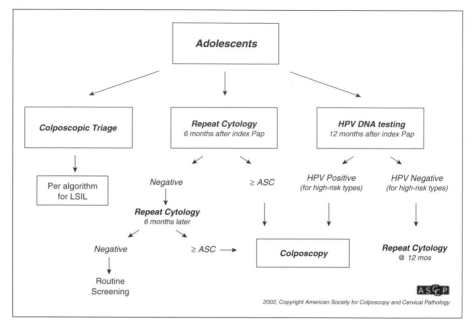

Figure 42-5 Management of women with low-grade squamous intraepithelial lesions in special circumstances. The Consensus Guidelines algorithms originally appeared in and are reprinted from *The Journal of Lower Genital Tract Disease*, Volume 16, issue 2, and are reprinted with the permission of ASCCP. © American Society for Colposcopy and Cervical Pathology 2002. No copies of the algorithms may be made without the prior consent of ASCCP

Follow up after excisional/ablative procedure if margins clear and no *in situ* cancer diagnosed: Literature is sparse but some authors (in the adult literature) recommend colposcopy at 4–6 months with follow up Pap tests every 4–6 months with or without HPV typing until at least three negative cytologic results and then return to routine Pap testing; if HPV testing is used and is negative can return to routine Pap testing

COLPOSCOPY PROCEDURE

Pregnancy test

Cervical sexually transmitted disease (STD) cultures

3–5% acetic acid to cervix for two minutes

Lugol's solution if no cervical lesion or vaginal lesion identified

Directed cervical/vaginal biopsies

ECC

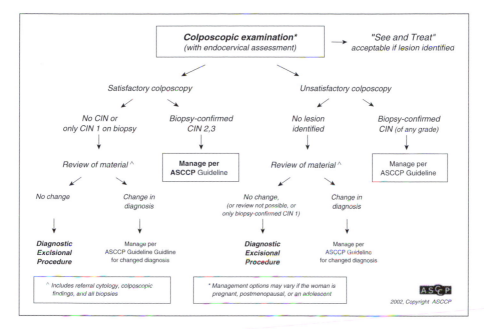

Figure 42-6   Management of women with high-grade squamous intraepithelial lesions (HSIL). The Consensus Guidelines algorithms originally appeared in and are reprinted from *The Journal of Lower Genital Tract Disease*, Volume 16, issue 2, and are reprinted with the permission of ASCCP. © American Society for Colposcopy and Cervical Pathology 2002. No copies of the algorithms may be made without the prior consent of ASCCP

LEEP PROCEDURE (EXCISIONAL)

Office/outpatient surgery procedure with intravenous sedation

Medium to large Grave's laser coated speculum

Lugol solution to cervix

Paracervical and intracervical block with 1% lidocaine without and with epinephrine, respectively

Loop selection based on the size of the lesion as above

One pass through lesion done on the cut setting (Move in perpendicular to lesion, come across beneath lesion, completed with an out perpendicular motion. Repeat pass(es) to remove the entire lesion as indicated (Use a 5 mm depth for CIN 2; 8–10 mm for CIN 3)

ECC

Edges first and then the bed of the cervix (with protection of cervical os) treated on cautery with the roller ball.

Once hemostasis is obtained, optional to place a fine layer of Monsel's solution

Nothing per vagina for 8–10 weeks

Table 42-2 Synopsis of management guidelines for biopsy-confirmed CIN

	Strength	Quality	Terminology
Women with biopsy-confirmed CIN-1			
When colposcopy is satisfactory:			
Options are follow-up without treatment or treatment using ablative or excisional modalities.			
Follow-up without treatment:			
Follow-up with repeat Pap test at 6 and 12 mo *or* HPV testing at 12 mo is preferred.	A	II	Preferred
Refer to colposcopy if repeat cytology of ASC or high-risk HPV DNA positive.	A	II	Preferred
After 2 negative cytology results or a negative HPV test, return to annual screening.	B	II	Preferred
A combination of repeat cytology and colposcopy at 12 mo is also acceptable for follow-up.	A	II	Acceptable
It is recommended that women with regression during follow-up repeat cytology at 12 mo.	B	III	Recommended
Decision to treat persistent CIN-1 should be based on patient and provider preferences.	B	III	
Treatment:			
Cryotherapy, laser ablation, and LEEP are all acceptable treatment modalities.	A	I	Acceptable
Treatment modality should be determined by the judgment of the clinician.	A	I	
Endocervical sampling is recommended before ablation of CIN-1.	A	II	Recommended
Excisional modalities are preferred for recurrent CIN-1 occurring after previous ablative therapy.	B	II	Preferred
When colposcopy is unsatisfactory:			
The preferred treatment is a diagnostic excisional procedure.	A	II	Preferred
Follow-up is acceptable in pregnant, immuno-suppressed women, and adolescent women.	C	III	Acceptable
Women with biopsy-confirmed CIN-2,3			
Initial management:			
Both excision and ablation are acceptable for women with CIN-2,3 and a satisfactory colposcopy.	A	I	Acceptable
In patients with recurrent CIN-2,3 excisional modalities are preferred.	A	II	Preferred
Diagnostic excisional procedures are recommended for CIN-2,3 and unsatisfactory colposcopy.	A	II	Recommended
Observation of CIN-2,3 with sequential cytology and colposcopy is unacceptable, except in special circumstances.	E	II	Unacceptable
Hysterectomy is unacceptable as primary therapy for CIN-2,3:	E	II	Unacceptable

(Continued)

Table 42-2 (*Continued*)

	Strength	Quality	Terminology
Follow-up after treatment:			
Follow-up using either cytology or combination of cytology and colposcopy at 4- to 6-mo intervals until at least 3 cytologic results are negative is acceptable.	A	II	Acceptable
During cytologic follow-up, the recommended threshold for referral to colposcopy is ASC.	A	II	Recommended
Annual cytology follow-up is recommended after 3 negative cytologic results are obtained.	A	II	Recommended
HPV DNA testing performed at least 6 mo after treatment is acceptable for surveillance.	B	II	Acceptable
If high-risk types of HPV are identified, colposcopy is recommended.	B	III	Recommended
If HPV testing is negative, triage to annual cytology follow-up is recommended.	B	II	Recommended
Repeat conization or hysterectomy based on a single positive HPV test is unacceptable.	D	III	Unacceptable
If CIN is identified at the margins of a diagnostic excisional procedure or in a postprocedure endocervical sampling.			
A colposcopic examination and an endocervical sampling is preferred at the 4- to 6-mo follow-up.	B	II	Preferred
A repeat diagnostic excisional procedure is acceptable in this setting.	A	II	Acceptable
Hysterectomy is acceptable in this situation when a repeat diagnostic excision is not feasible.	B	II	Acceptable

Used with permission from: Wright TC, Cox JT, Massad LS, *et al.* 2001 Consensus guidelines for the management of women with cervical intraepithelial neoplasia. *Am J Obstet Gynecol* 2003:189;295–304

Strength of recommendation: A, Good evidence for efficacy and substantial clinical benefit support recommendation for use; B, Moderate evidence for efficacy or only limited clinical benefit supports recommendation for use; C, Evidence for efficacy is insufficient to support a recommendation for or against use, but recommendations may be made on other grounds; D, Moderate evidence for lack of efficacy or for adverse outcome supports a recommendation against use; E, Good evidence for lack of efficacy or for adverse outcome supports a recommendation against use.

Quality of evidence: I, Evidence from at least 1 randomized, controlled trial; II, Evidence from at least 1 clinical trial without randomization, from cohort or case-controlled analytic studies (preferably from more than 1 center), or from multiple time-series studies, or dramatic results from uncontrolled experiments; III, Evidence from opinions of respected authorities based on clinical experience, descriptive studies, or reports of expert committees.

Terminology: Recommended, Good data to support use when only 1 option is available; Preferred, Option is the best (or 1 of the best) when there are multiple other options; Acceptable, One of multiple options when there are either data indicating that another approach is superior or when there are no data to favor any single option; Unacceptable, Good data against use.

CRYOTHERAPY PROCEDURE (ABLATIVE)[†]

Identify lesion colposcopically

Select cryo probe that is correct size to cover lesion

Apply lubricant (e.g. KY jelly) to probe

Use freeze–thaw–freeze technique: cervix is frozen for 3 minutes, allowed to thaw for 5 minutes and frozen again for 3 minutes

Care should be taken to protect the vagina during the procedure to avoid freezing vaginal sidewalls

[†]Cryotherapy while reported in the literature to be equally effective is more operator-dependent

VULVAR INTRAEPITHELIAL NEOPLASIA (VIN)

Management

Biopsy proven VIN 1–3:

Imiquimod (Aldara Cream, 3M Pharmaceuticals, St. Paul, MN) 5% up to three times a week (if skin shows evidence of erosion from cream try once a week then increase to twice a week) for four months; rebiopsy, if VIN 2 or more persists consider laser treatment (see below for VIN 3) and/or referral to gynecology oncology for treatment and follow-up

Biopsy proven VIN 3:

Superficial laser ablation followed by silvadene cream to heal; once healed Imiquimod 5% up to three times a week as skin tolerates for four months; rebiopsy. If VIN 1 or less just observe yearly with Pap tests

VAGINAL INTRAEPITHELIAL NEOPLASIA (VAIN)

Management

Biopsy proven VAIN 1:

Early research studies with Imiquimod 5% in adults; none in adolescents

Biopsy proven VAIN 2–3:

CO_2 laser is the standard treatment

BIBLIOGRAPHY

www.asccp.org/consensus/cytological (ASCCP 2002 Algorithms for Management of Women With Abnormal Cervical Cytology)

www.cancer.org (American Cancer Society Detection Guidelines 2002)

The ASCUS-LSIL Triage Study (ALTS) Group. Results of a randomized trial on the management of cytology interpretations of atypical squamous cells of undetermined significance. *Am J Obstet Gynecol* 2003;188:1383–92

The ASCUS-LSIL Triage Study (ALTS) Group. A randomized trial on the management of low-grade squamous intraepithelial lesion cytology interpretations. *Am J Obstet Gynecol* 2003;188:1393–400

Cox T, Schiffman M, Solomon D. Prospective follow-up suggests similar risk of subsequent cervical intraepithelial neoplasia grade 2 or 3 among women with cervical inrtraepithelial neoplasia grade 1 or negative colposcopy and directed biopsy. *Am J Obstet Gynecol* 2003;188:1406–13

Diakomanolis G, Haidopoulos D, Stefanidis K. Treatment of high grade vaginal intraepithelial neoplasia with Imiquimod cream (Letter). *N Engl J Med* 2002;347:374

Guido R, Schiffman M, Solomon D, *et al*. Postcolposcopy management strategies for women referred with low grade squamous intraepithelial lesion or human papillomavirus DNA-positive atypical squamous cells of undetermined significance: a two-year prospective study. *Am J Obstet Gynecol* 2003;188:1401–5

Jayne CJ, Kaufman RH. Treatment of vulvar intraepithelial neoplasia 2/3 with Imiquimod cream. *J Reprod Med* 2002;47:395–8

Kahn JA, Hillard PJ. Cervical cytology screening and management of abnormal cytology in adolescent girls. *J Pediatr Adolesc Gynecol* 2003;16:167–71

Mitchell MF, Tortelero-Luna G, Cook E, *et al*. A randomized clinical trial of cryotherapy, laser vaporization and loop electrical excision for the treatment of squamous intraepithelial lesions of the cervix. *Obstet Gynecol* 1998;92:737–44

Solomon D, Davey D, Kurman R, *et al*. The 2001 Bethesda System: terminology for reporting results of cervical cytology. *J Am Med Assoc* 2002;287:2114–9

Wright TC, Cox JT, Massad LS, *et al*. 2001 Consensus guidelines for the management of women with cervical cytological abnormalities. *J Am Med Assoc* 2002;287:2120–9

Wright TC, Cox JT, Massad LS, *et al*. 2001 Consensus guidelines for the management of women with cervical intraepithelial neoplasia. *Am J Obstet Gynecol* 2003;189:295–304

43 Pelvic inflammatory disease (PID)

Ascending polymicrobial genital tract infection that occurs in sexually active females

Includes array of inflammatory disorders: endometritis, parametritis, salpingitis, oophoritis, tubo-ovarian abscess (TOA), peritonitis, and perihepatitis

Neisseria gonorrhoeae (GC) and *Chlamydia trachomatis* (CT) are usually the causative agents but microflora from the vagina and bowel may also contribute

Serious medical and social consequences: chronic pain, ectopic pregnancy and infertility

DIAGNOSIS

Surgical

Gold standard is laparoscopy but should only be utilized in:

A sick patient with high suspicion of a competing diagnosis (i.e. appendicitis)

An acutely ill patient who has failed outpatient treatment for PID

Any patient not clearly improving after approximately 72 h of inpatient treatment for PID

Clinical

Positive predictive value of clinical diagnosis when compared to surgical diagnosis ranges from 65–90%

Risk factors for PID

Age 14–24

Sexually active

Multiple sex partners

New sex partner

History of sexually transmitted disease (STD)

History of PID

Use of an intrauterine device (IUD)

Pelvic instrumentation

Nulliparity

Onset of pelvic/abdominal pain within 1 week of menses; tubo-ovarian abscess more likely if pain presents more than 18 days after menses

CDC (2002) criteria for clinical diagnosis of PID

Minimum:

Uterine/adnexal tenderness *or*

Cervical motion tenderness

Additional criteria useful in the diagnosis

Oral temp > 101°F (> 38.3°C)

Abnormal cervical or vaginal discharge

Elevated erythrocyte sedimentation rate (ESR) or C-reactive protein (CRP)

Evidence of cervical infection with GC or CT

White blood cells on saline microscopy

Definitive diagnostic criteria:

Endometrial biopsy showing histopathologic evidence of endometritis

Transvaginal ultrasound or MRI showing thick fluid filled tubes; TOA, a discrete cystic or complex mass with internal echoes

Laparoscopic abnormalities consistent with PID

Criteria for hospital admission:

Failure of oral treatment

Inability of patient to follow or tolerate oral regimen

Inability to exclude surgical emergency

Pregnancy

Severe illness, nausea, vomiting, or high fever

TOA

MANAGEMENT

See Figure 43-1

Treatment

In-patient

Parenteral Regimen A:

Cefoxitin sodium 2 g IV q 6 h *or*

Cefotetan disodium 2 g IV q 12 h

plus

Doxycycline 100 mg IV/po q 12 h

after discharge, the patient continues doxycycline 100 mg po bid for total of 14 days of treatment

Parenteral Regimen B:

Clindamycin 900 mg IV q 8 hr

plus

Gentamicin IV/IM (loading dose of 2 mg/kg of body weight followed by a maintenance dose of 1.5 mg/kg q 8 h). Single daily dosing may be substituted

After discharge, the patient continues doxycycline 100 mg po bid or clindamycin 450 mg po qid for a total of 14 days of treatment

Clinical experience should guide decision regarding transition to oral therapy

No objective findings: fever, leukocytosis or enlarging TOA

Decreasing symptoms

Twenty-four hours or more of IV antibiotics

Tuboovarian abscess (TOA)

Usually treat with IV antibiotics for 7 days then oral clindamycin 450 mg qid for at least 7 more days or until abscess gone by transabdominal ultrasound; warning signs for *Clostridium difficile*

If no improvement or worsening within 48 h by nature of persistent high fever, increasing size of abscess, persistently high level of leukocytosis – Add ampicillin 2 g IV every 4 h; if no improvement or worsening in 48 h then surgical evaluation

Conservative management surgically:

- Laparoscopy: incision and drainage of abscess; irrigate with copious saline

- Percutaneous (anterior abdomen, posterior transgluteal, transvaginal) drainage guided by CT or ultrasound (consult with radiology)

- If unsuccessful, remove as little ovarian tissue as needed

Out-patient treatment guidelines (do not use unless compliance can be guaranteed)

Regimen A (Quinolones can be used in child < 18 years if > 45 kg):

Ofloxacin 400 mg bid for 14 days *or*

Levofloxacin 500 mg qd for 14 days

with or without

Metronidazole 500 mg bid for 14 days

Regimen B:

Cefoxitin 2 g IM; plus Probenecid (Mylan Pharmaceuticals Inc., Morgantown, WV), 1 g po concurrently *or*

Ceftriaxone (Rocephin, Roche Pharmaceuticals, Nutley, NJ) 250 mg IM

plus

Doxycycline 100 mg po bid for 14 days

with or without

Metronidazole 500 mg po bid for 14 days

Adjunct treatment

Evaluation for pregnancy, other STDs (HIV, syphilis, hepatitis B), substance abuse when indicated should be performed upon admission or at out-patient visit

Hospital Admission Orders
Pelvic Inflammatory Disease (PID)
MD to check yes or no or where indicated
All statements are to be considered standing orders

Date/Time

Pelvic Inflammatory Disease   Weight _____
  Patients > 45 kg   Height _____

Admission criteria include abdominal pain and:

a) uterine/adnexal tenderness and/or
b) cervical motion tenderness (if no other cause for illness found)

Additional admission criteria (not required)

  a)   oral temperature of >101F (>38.3 C)
  b)   abnormal cervical or microprurulent discharge
  c)   presence of white blood cells (WBC) on saline microscopy of vaginal secretions (wet prep)
  d)   elevated C-reactive protein (CRP)
  e)   laboratory documentation of cervical infection with *N. gonorrhea* (GC) or *C. Trachomatis* (CT)

PHYSICIAN'S ORDERS:
1. Admit Dr. _____   Criteria at end of order sheet
   Place in 23 hrs. observation Dr. _____
2. Diagnosis Uncomplicated Pelvic Inflammatory
   Disease _____ _____
3. Condition Good Fair Poor
4. Allergies _____
5. Diet _____
6. Vital Signs _____
7. Activity
8. Diagnostic tests (if not done in Emergency Department)
   Pregnancy test
   Clean catch U/A and C/S
   CBC with diff
   GC & CT amplification swab of cervix   If GC and/or CT positive, check
   CRP   hepatitis B & HIV serologies
   RPR
  Transvaginal US if temperature greater than
  101, elevated WBC, or inadequate pelvic
  exam prior to starting antibx
9. Antibiotics (Select one group)
   Cefotetan 2 g IV q 12° (adult dose)
   or
   Doxycycline 100 mg IV q 12° (adult dose)   Bioavailability similar unless
                                             contraindicated give po
   or
   Doxycycline 100 mg po q 12°
   OR
  Clindamycin 900 mg IV q 8° (adult dose)   Preferred for tubo-ovarian abscess.
   Gentamicin_____ mg (2 mg/kg) IV loading dose   7 days single IV daily dose may be
   Then Gentamicin_____ mg (1.5 mg/kg)   substituted
   Iv q 8° (adult dose)

                    M.D. Signature _____ Date _____

Figure 43.1   PID clinical pathway

Hospital Admission Orders
Pelvic Inflammatory Disease (PID)
MD to check yes or no or where indicated
All statements are to be considered standing orders

10. _____ @ _____ cc/hr
    Type of IV fluids   Rate

May decrease after 24° or patient
improves with no fever, minimal
abdominal pain/tenderness,
no elevation WBC and willing
to comply with outpatient
treatment

11. Consults
   Social Services
   GYN reconsult

If no improvement in 72 hours,
reconsult

Discharge Criteria
   No fever
   Minimal abdominal pain/tenderness
   WBC not elevated
   Willing to comply with outpatient treatment

Discharge Antibiotics (Complete 14 day course)
   Doxycycline 100 mg po BID x _____ days
OR
   Metronidazole 500 mg TID x _____ days
   and
   Doxycycline 100 mg q 12º x _____ days
   or
   Clindamycin 450 mg po qid x _____ days

If tubo-ovarian abscess suspected

Contraception
(List choices) _____

Provide teaching session on sexually
transmitted diseases, contraception
methods and condom directions
for use

Followup
Teen Pregnancy Prevention Clinic:

on _____ at _____

Should have demonstrated plan with
guardian/adult for obtaining
outpatient medications

Your primary medical doctor:

Dr. _____ on _____ at _____

Pediatric Gynecology:

on _____ at _____

M.D. Signature _____ Date _____

Check if Present _____

Education needs to be given with either in- or out-patient treatment

    Education about STDs, PID etiology, prevention, course

    Education about hepatitis B immunization (if not completed)

    Education about contraception

Social service evaluation to assess family, school performance, psychologic status

Follow-up

Follow-up examination for out-patient regimen at 48–72 h after initiation to assure improvement. If no improvement or worsening, admit for intravenous antibiotics and further evaluation, including ultrasound if not done prior

Follow-up examination for either regimen at two weeks after initiation to assess improvement and then at 4–6 weeks after treatment for screening for reinfection with *Chlamydia* and *Gonorrhea* (if not done within a year). Nothing per vagina recommended until 8 week visit. At that visit, social issues should be readdressed, contraceptive compliance should be assessed, and knowledge base regarding STDs and PID should be reinforced

BIBLIOGAPHY

Sexually Transmitted Diseases Treatment Guidelines 2002. *MMWR* 2002;51(RR-6) CDC website: http://www.cdc.gov/mmwr

44 Pelvic pain

ACUTE PELVIC PAIN

KEY POINTS

The differential diagnosis for acute pelvic pain is long/varied

The common gynecologic causes include infection, ovarian cysts, endometriosis, ectopic pregnancy, adnexal torsion or musculoskeletal pathology

Non-gynecologic causes involve gastrointestinal, urinary, neurologic, or less commonly psychologic causes

DIFFERENTIAL DIAGNOSIS

Gynecologic
Pregnancy-related
    Ectopic pregnancy
    Threatened abortion
Ovarian causes
    Cyst/mass
    Torsion

Fallopian tube
    Torsion
Infection
    Endometritis
    Pelvic inflammatory disease
Cyclic
    Mittleschmerz
    Dysmenorrhea
    Endometriosis
    Obstructive mullerian anomalies

Non-gynecologic
Gastrointestinal
    Appendicitis
    Gastroenteritis
    Inflammatory bowel disease
    Gallstones

Genitourinary
    Nephrolithiasis
    Urinary tract infection
    Pyelonephritis
Musculoskeletal
    Acute iliopsoas muscle spasm
Neurologic
    Nerve entrapment
Psychologic
    History of sexual abuse
    Psychosomatic

DIAGNOSIS

History

When did the pain begin? (What is proximity to last menstrual period?)

Location of pain (R or LLQ, periumbilical, etc)

Nature of pain (sharp, crampy, stabbing, constant, intermittent)

Radiation (to back, down legs)

Relieving/exacerbating symptoms

- Walking/exercise/eating/urinating/bowel movement

Associated symptoms

- Nausea, vomiting, fever, diarrhea, dysuria

Gynecologic history

- Menarche, when pain occurred in relationship to menarche?
- Sexual/contraceptive history?
- Could patient be pregnant?

Historical clues:

Mittelschmerz:	Ovulatory pain, typically dull pain at time of ovulation lasting few minutes to 6–8 hours (can be treated with non-steroidal antiinflammatory drugs or oral contraceptives)
Dysmenorrhea:	Pain with menses, could even have nausea, vomiting, diarrhea
Torsion:	Sudden onset of pain, typically followed closely by nausea vs appendicitis with gradual onset of pain, more periumbilical at first with later onset of nausea and/or anorexia
Musculoskeletal:	Burning pain that is worse with movement, better with rest
	Can involve low back pain, could be worse with menses
	No associated fever, increased white blood cell count (WBC)

Physical examination

Complete physical exam with vital signs

Close attention to abdominal exam:

- Assess for presence of masses, tenderness, hepatosplenomegaly, hernia, peritoneal signs
- Assess for iliospoas tenderness (see Chronic pelvic pain)

Check back for:

- Costovertebral angle (CVA) tenderness/muscle pain

Pelvic:

- Ensure a patent vaginal opening
- If able to use speculum:

  Evaluate vaginal walls for bulging from an obstructive anomaly

  Obtain endocervical testing for chlamydia and gonorrhea

- Bimanual vaginal-abdominal, rectoabdominal or rectovaginal-abdominal exam (single digit exam preferred):

  Assess size, tenderness of uterus

  Presence of cervical motion tenderness

  Presence of adnexal mass or tenderness

  Ensure patient not impacted with stool; heme test stool

Laboratory testing (base on assessment)

Complete blood count (CBC)

Erythrocyte sedimentation rate (ESR)

Urinalysis

Urine culture

Cervical cultures

Pregnancy test

Stool for occult blood

Imaging

Pelvic ultrasound:

- IF palpate pelvic/adnexal mass
- IF adequate pelvic not possible

Gastrointestinal films/skeletal films/other tests:

- As indicated by history
- Spiral CT can help rule in or out appendicitis but may not delineate pelvic organs well

Management

Based on etiology

When diagnosis in question:

- Diagnostic laparoscopy may help delineate cause by visualizing the pelvic organs, appendix, liver and gallbladder

CHRONIC PELVIC PAIN (CPP)

KEY POINTS

Endometriosis and musculoskeletal causes are the most common etiologies in the female adolescent

DEFINITION

Lower abdominal menstrual or non-menstrual pain of at least 6 months duration

COMMON CAUSES

Endometriosis

Myofascial pain

Pelvic adhesions

Pelvic inflammatory disease

Irritable bowel syndrome

DIAGNOSIS

Assess for the five major sources that might contribute to CPP:

	Cyclic	*Non-cyclic*
Gynecologic	Dysmenorrhea	Endometriosis
	Mittelschmerz	Ovarian mass
	Endometriosis	Adhesions
	Obstructive mullerian anomalies	

Musculoskeletal	Musculoskeletal causes	Musculoskeletal
Gastrointestinal		Irritable bowel
		Inflammatory bowel
		Lactose intolerance
Urologic		
Psychological		

History

When was pain first noted

Localize pain – groin, back, abdomen (R, L, upper, lower, umbilical), buttock, leg

Radiation (does or does not?)

Is pain hormonally responsive?

- Cyclic or premenstrual?

Characterize pain:

- Burning sensation – indicates muscular component
- Sharp, stabbing, aching, squeezing, throbbing

Pain is worse at what time

Pain is worse with what activity

Pain is better with what position, activity

Does the pain awaken you from sleep?/Can you sleep if you are in pain?

Any associated symptoms: nausea, vomiting, dysuria, dyschezia

What pain medicines used

ROS:	Bowel disease	
	Constipation:	Frequency of stooling/Do you feel completely empty after stooling?
	Irritable bowel syndrome:	Not easily diagnosed in adolescent Adult symptoms:
		Irregular stooling pattern
		Constipation alternating with diarrhea
		Pain relieved with defecation
		Abdominal distention
		Passage of mucus

Inflammatory bowel disease	ulcerative colitis: tenesmus/explosive diarrhea
	Crohn's disease: dull, chronic lower abdominal pain
Urinary tract disease:	Urinary tract infections, dysuria, frequency

Substance use

Depression

Sexual/physical/psychological abuse

Physical examination

Note: Need a complete exam, the sequence of which is important, save the bimanual for the final step as it incorporates many levels of tissue (e.g. uterus as well as abdominal musculature)

Observe posture of patient during interview, walking to exam, self-selected posture

- Look for evidence of lordosis, one-legged standing, leg-length discrepancy
- Palpate lower back for pain

Abdomen:

- Have patient identify area of tenderness and avoid that area at first
- Try to locate any trigger points
- Skin: With patient in supine position start at epigastric region and run fingers perpendicular to rectus muscle from epigastric area to pubic bone

  Tell patient to identify any area of tenderness along rectus

  If located, have patient lift head – IF worsens, pain may be an abdominal trigger point

- Psoas muscle: At level of umbilicus, move lateral to rectus and press down into psoas muscle. IF tender, have patient perform ipsilateral straight leg lift, IF worsens pain – psoas trigger point identified

- Iliacus muscle: At anterior superior iliac spine, curve fingertips into iliacus muscle, IF tender have patient perform ipsilateral straight leg lift (keep knee locked and straight while elevating leg off exam table). IF tenderness worses – Iliacus trigger point of iliospoas identified

- Palpate each quadrant of abdomen for tenderness/masses
- Evaluate for hepatosplenomegaly/hernias

Pelvic exam:

- Perform single digit exam of vagina
- Palpate urethra, palpate lateral sidewalls of vagina (at 5 and 8 o'clock) to locate any levator muscle trigger point/tenderness
- Check uterosacral ligaments
- Check position/shape/mobility/tenderness of uterus
- Speculum exam
    - Pap smear/sexually transmitted disease (STD) testing as indicated
- Bimanual exam – this part of exam compresses muscles and genitourinary organs together confounding exam – assess for uterine enlargement, adnexal masses
- Rectal exam – heme test stool

Laboratory

Complete blood count – look for inflammation

Urinalysis – evaluate for renal disease

STD testing

Erythrocyte sedimentation rate (ESR) – check for inflammation/inflammatory bowel disease

Human chorionic gonadotropin (hCG) – rule out pregnancy

Imaging

Pelvic ultrasound: Rule out pelvic mass/utero-ovarian pathology

Plain abdominal film: Rule out constipation

Diagnostic laparoscopy

MANAGEMENT

Two possible approaches:

(1) Empiric method – Sequentially prescribe drug treatments for most likely causes and involve multidisciplinary evaluation (urology, gastrointestinal (GI), physical therapy)

- IF treatment relieves the pain, one can presume underlying cause and claim therapeutic success. IF not proceed with laparoscopy

Diagnostic laparoscopy:

- Indications: Progressive dysmenorrhea without response to NSAIDs/OCPs either in cyclic or continuous therapy, failed other hormonal methods (e.g. Depo-Provera)

  Suspected ovarian or uterine abnormalities

  Unexplained painful, irregular bleeding

  Cases of diagnostic quandary

- Look for evidence of endometriosis

  Appearance not always the typical powder-burn spots of adults (see Endometriosis, Chapter 18)

(2) Diagnostic method – Intensive diagnostic testing and include laparoscopy as part of initial workup (indications as above)

Treatment

Primary dysmenorrhea:	Painful menses in absence of specific pathologic cause
Secondary dysmenorrhea:	Painful menses due to specific gynecologic condition (e.g. endometriosis, obstructive mullerian anomalies)
	See Dysmenorrhea (Chapter 14) for treatment
Endometriosis:	See Endometriosis (Chapter 18) for treatment
	Base treatment on severity of pain/ preservation of anatomy and response to previous treatment
	Surgical treatment (ablation/excision)
	Medical treatment
	OCPs/Depo-Provera/GnRH analogues
GI symptoms/increased ESR:	Consider gastroenterology referral to work-up for inflammatory bowel disease or other GI etiology
Urinary tract disease:	Urologic referral

If pain worse with movement/better with rest, and/or identify muscle spasm/trigger point on exam and suspect musculoskeletal pain:

> Refer to physical therapy (PT)
>
> Even in cases of uncertain etiology or significant pathology, i.e. dysmenorrhea, endometriosis, a musculoskeletal component may be present and a PT referral might be helpful

45 Polycystic ovarian syndrome (PCOS)

Also called hyperandrogenic chronic anovulation (HCA)

Many women with PCOS have onset of symptoms during adolescence

PCOS is the most common cause of hyperandrogenism/hirsutism in adolescent girls

Preadolescent girls with idiopathic premature adrenarche are at risk of PCOS

Patients may be thin, normal or obese in size

DEFINITION

A clinical syndrome of:

- Ovulatory dysfunction
- Clinical evidence of hyperandrogenism and/or hyperandrogenemia (hirsutism, acne, androgenic alopecia)
- Exclusion of related disorders (hyperprolactinemia, thyroid disorders, non-classical congenital adrenal hyperplasia (CAH))

PATHOPHYSIOLOGY

Basic defect is inappropriate gonadotropin (FSH, LH) stimulation of the ovary by the hypothalamic–pituitary unit. Without proper signaling to the ovary, multiple small immature follicles (cysts) are present, hence the term 'polycystic ovary'. This typical ovarian appearance is uncommonly seen in the adolescent

A secondary defect is insulin resistance

PRESENTATION

Characteristic history of irregular menses with or without associated hirsutism/acne (see Hirsutism, Chapter 24)

May have had a history of premature adrenarche

Patients with delayed onset of menses (> 2 years between onset of secondary sexual characteristics and menses)

Obese patients with oligomenorrhea (also at increased risk of diabetes)

Obesity and hirsutism that predate menarche

Uncommonly, adolescents can develop virilization (see Hirsutism, Chapter 24)

DIAGNOSIS

History

Menstrual pattern

Hirsutism (location, rapidity of onset, previous treatments, family history)

Acne

Weight changes

Family history: diabetes, gestational diabetes

Physical examination

Weight: majority of patients are overweight but some may be thin. Upper body obesity common and defined as waist to hip ratio > 0.85

Blood pressure (BP): Rule out hypertension, elevations in BP may be due to CAH or obesity

Skin:

Assess hirsutism, use Ferriman–Gallwey scoring (see Hirsutism, Chapter 24)

Look for acanthosis nigricans – velvety, hyperpigmented, verrucous skin in the nape of neck, axilla, under breasts, in vulva and other body folds: associated with hyperinsulinemia

Body habitus: look for stigmata of Cushing's – striae, buffalo-hump

Thyroid: look for enlargement

Abdomen:

> Look for male escutcheon

> Assess for abdominal masses

External genitalia:

> Look for clitoromegaly

> Assess for signs of estrogenization: With severe hyperandrogenism, estrogen levels will be suppressed

> Rule out other causes of anovulation (see Dysfunctional uterine bleeding, Chapter 13)

Laboratory tests

Check FSH, TSH, prolactin levels and prescribe Provera 10 mg po × 10 days

> If FSH, TSH, prolactin are normal and patient has withdrawal bleed:

>> Diagnosis: PCOS

If patient hirsute, additional tests necessary:

> Check total testosterone

>> Should be less than 150 ng/dl

>> If > 100 ng/dl – rule out ovarian tumor with ultrasound

> Check 7 am 17-hydroxyprogesterone acetate level

>> If < 100 ng/dl, normal

>> IF 100–300 ng/dl, perform adrenocorticotropic hormone (ACTH) stimulation test

>> - To rule out CAH

>> IF > 300 ng/dl, diagnosis likely CAH

> Check dehydroepiandrosterone sulfate (DHEAS)

>> If > 700 ng/dl, rule out adrenal cause with CT of adrenals

>> - (see CAH)

> Check fasting insulin/glucose:

>> If family history of diabetes

>> If patient's mother had gestational diabetes

>> If acanthosis nigricans/obesity noted on physical exam

>> IF ratio glucose/insulin < 4.5, consider therapy for insulin resistance (see below)

MANAGEMENT

Goals

(1) Hormonal suppression to lower ovarian androgens, improve acne and hirsutism, prevent chronic estrogen exposure to the endometrium and thereby prevent endometrial hyperplasia/carcinoma

  • Mechanism of action: Estrogens increase sex hormone binding globulin, decrease free testosterone and decrease production of adrenal androgens

(2) To address issue of hyperinsulinemia

Treatment options

If irregular menstruation:

Cyclic progestins:

  Provera 10 mg po cycle days 1–14 of the month *or*

  Cyclic oral contraceptives

If hirsute:

  Add antiandrogen

    Spironolactone 100 mg po bid

    May not see decrease in hair for 3–6 months

  Consider adjunctive hair treatments:

    Waxing, bleaching, electrolysis, laser removal

If insulin resistant and obese:

  Strict caloric restriction (1500 kcal/day)

  Aerobic exercise

  Consider use of insulin potentiating medications. May need referral to endocrinology for this:

  • Metformin (Glucophage®)

    Start 500 mg po bid for one week then tid

    Draw baseline electrolytes, creatinine, lactate dehydrogenase

    Then follow every 8 weeks

  • Use is associated with risk of lactic acidosis

- Must temporarily discontinue use with dehydration/use of intravenous dyes as with radiographic studies until rehydrated and renal function recovers
- Use contraindicated with renal insufficiency, congestive heart failure, hepatic dysfunction, metabolic acidosis, surgery, alcohol use

Long term counseling:

PCOS patients at risk of:

Abnormal glucose metabolism

Type II diabetes mellitus

Dyslipidemia

- Emphasize weight reduction, e.g. weight watchers
- Emphasize exercise
- Assess for self-image issues and provide referral to psychotherapy as needed (see Depression, Chapter 12)

BIBLIOGRAPHY

Kahn JA, Gordon CM. Polycystic ovary syndrome. *Adolesc Med State of the Art Rev* 1999;10:321–36.

Stafford DEJ, Gordon CM. Adolescent androgen abnormalities. *Curr Opin Obstet Gynecol* 2002;14:445–51

46 Pregnancy

Maternal and neonatal complications increased in pregnant adolescents under the age of 17:

Triple the adult neonatal death rate (within 28 days of birth)

Double the adult maternal death rate

Other: poor maternal weight gain, prematurity, pregnancy-induced hypertension, anemia, and sexually transmitted diseases (STDs)

Recent studies suggest pregnant adolescents under the age of 15 may have even higher risks

Psychosocial complications:

For the mother: school interruption, persistent poverty, limited vocational opportunities, separation from the child's father, divorce and repeat pregnancy

For the child: increased neglect, developmental delay, academic difficulties, behavioral disorders, substance abuse, adolescent parent

For the father: poor academic performance, limited financial resources, reduced income potential

Research suggests that comprehensive adolescent pregnancy programs contribute to prevention of psychosocial complications and promotion of good outcomes

DIAGNOSIS

Clinical suspicion and/or menstrual abnormalities

Check beta subunit of human chorionic gonadotropin (βhCG)

History

(Alone with adolescent more likely to ensure honesty)

Menstrual history:

- When was your last and the previous menstrual period? Were they normal?
- Do you engage in sexual activity?
- Do you use contraception?
- Is there any chance you may be pregnant?
- What would you do if a pregnancy test is positive?

    While the rate of suicide is low in pregnancy, if the teen does respond that she may endanger herself, immediate psychiatric evaluation is essential

    A discussion of how a teen would respond to the reality of pregnancy or motherhood before the test is performed helps to facilitate abstract thinking as well as pregnancy prevention

Physical examination

Look for signs of pregnancy:

Breast exam: engorged breasts with darkening of the areola

Abdominal exam: tenderness or enlargement

Pelvic exam should be performed (see Gynecologic examination, Chapter 21) with cervical STD cultures: bluish cervix (Chadwick's sign)

Bimanual exam: pelvic tenderness; uterine enlargement

- Uterus remains a pelvic organ until 12 weeks gestation when it becomes sufficiently large to palpate abdominally just above the symphysis pubis; at 16 weeks, the uterine fundus is palpable midway between the symphysis and umbilicus; at 20 weeks the uterine fundus is palpable at umbilicus
- If uterus does not seem enlarged and there is adnexal tenderness and/or enlargement the diagnosis of ectopic pregnancy must be ruled out (see below)

Laboratory tests

A clinical diagnosis of pregnancy must be confirmed by laboratory testing:

Urine pregnancy test (UCG): the most common method to confirm pregnancy

- Provides an accurate qualitative result (positive or negative) with hCG as low as 5–50 mIU/ml depending on the assay; should wait at least 14 days after a sexual experience to be certain
- Positive test does not exclude the possibility of an ectopic or non-viable intrauterine pregnancy
- If a pregnancy is suspected despite a negative test, test should be repeated in one week
- Severe renal disease with elevated lipids, high immunoglobin levels and low serum protein can interfere with test results
- If urine is too dilute the test results can be adversely affected
- An office-based test should be performed to confirm a home-based test result

Serum pregnancy test: qualitative or quantitative βhCG

- Qualitative hCG test reports presence or absence of hCG (lower limit of detectability varies with assay used)
- Quantitative hCG testing when uncertain will report the amount of hCG in the serum

   Serial quantitative test specimens can be obtained to check doubling time or disappearance time when ectopic pregnancy or an impending spontaneous abortion are being evaluated

- Pelvic ultrasound: helpful when an accurate gestational age or viability or location of a pregnancy also is being evaluated

   Transvaginal ultrasound:

      Gestational sac is usually visible at 4.5–5 weeks' gestation (hCG level 1500–3000 mIU/ml)

   Transabdominal ultrasound:

      Structures are noted slightly later

MANAGEMENT

Decision-making regarding outcome of pregnancy:

(1) After confirming pregnancy, inform the adolescent of the test result

- Elicit her thoughts and feelings about the test result
- Ambivalence, apathy, fear, tearfulness, or even shock should be anticipated
- Providing emotional support is **key**

(2) Find out how she wants to go about informing her parent(s) and the father of the baby

- Schedule another office visit if she is not able to inform her parents of the pregnancy
- Most adolescents inform their parents within this time period and on their own terms

(3) Provide factual information regarding estimated date of confinement (EDC) and prenatal care and course despite her initial plans

- Options regarding the pregnancy outcome should be discussed in a non-judgmental manner

(4) Should be referred to a physician or clinic where comprehensive pregnancy counseling is provided unless the care provider has expertise in pregnancy counseling

- All options (abortion, adoption, parenthood) should be discussed; knowledge of such resources is available through referrals from colleagues, women's clinics, and the phone directory
- Care provider should check in with the adolescent about one week after the scheduled referral for follow-up information to demonstrate concern for the adolescent and to ensure appropriate care

Adolescents choosing to terminate the pregnancy should be aware that some states require parental notification for a legal abortion only by the healthcare personnel performing the procedure

A judicial bypass system also exists if the judge determines that the adolescent is a mature minor or if termination of pregnancy is in the minor's best interest

No legal requirement to notify the father of the baby prior to the termination

Adolescents deciding to continue their pregnancies to term should be referred to specialized prenatal care as soon as possible:

Early testing for STDs, initiation of prenatal vitamins and good nutrition, and assessment of underlying familial and medical conditions

Early counseling regarding what to expect during the pregnancy, avoidance of substance abuse, prevention of STDs

Social Service assistance

Facilitate enrollment in prenatal care and with financial assistance

Facilitate continued education

IMMEDIATE REFERRAL TO A SPECIALIST

Adolescents with certain medical conditions are at increased risk for complications during pregnancy and early consultation with the specialist is recommended so those risks can be discussed with the adolescent:

- Diabetes mellitus
- Epilepsy
- Cardiac disease
- Sickle cell anemia and sickle trait
- Cancer
- Acne – on Accutane

PREGNANCY COMPLICATIONS

Bleeding or spotting occurs in 20–25% of pregnancies; approximately half of these pregnancies abort spontaneously; determine blood group and antibody status with prophylactic administration of anti-D gamma-globulin given to rhesus-negative patient

- Septic abortion: presence of fever, abdominal tenderness; emergent evaluation and treatment
- Threatened abortion: viable pregnancy; cervix closed; no treatment
- Incomplete abortion: cervical os is open; treatment is immediate suction D&C
- Complete abortion: cervical os is closed, ultrasound shows minimal tissue, minimal bleeding; expectant management
- Missed abortion: gestational sac/fetal pole without fetal heart motion on transvaginal ultrasound at 8 weeks gestation or with hCG 20 000 mIU/ml; scheduled suction D&C

Complaints of bleeding and/or abdominal pain: ectopic pregnancy until proven otherwise

- Quantitative hCG levels should approximately double over 48 hours
- If hCG is doubling appropriately, a gestational sac is visible in the uterine cavity by 1500–3000mIU/ml hCG level on transvaginal ultrasound
- If hCG not doubling or nothing in the uterus and adnexa normal by transvaginal ultrasound then a uterine curettage should demonstrate villi on pathology

- If not consider this an ectopic pregnancy (see Tubal mass, Chapter 59 for treatment)
- Abdominal pain can also be a common symptom of a normal gestation with/without a corpus luteal cyst; appendicitis can occur coincidentally with pregnancy
- Bleeding can represent cervicitis secondary to an STD

INTERNET RESOURCES

www.ferre.org/workbook
www.plannedparenthood.org

BIBLIOGRAPHY

Chacko MR. *Pregnancy in Adolescents*. Up To Date 2002;10(3)
Polaneczky M, O'Connor K. Pregnancy in the adolescent patient: screening, diagnosis, and initial management. Adolescent gynecology, part II: the sexually active adolescent. *Pediatr Clin North Am* 1999;46:649–63

47 Premature ovarian failure (POF)

DEFINITION

Amenorrhea due to ovarian failure prior to the age of 40 years old

Follicle stimulating hormone (FSH) level is in the menopausal range for the assay, typically > 30 IU/l

CLINICAL PRESENTATION

POF can occur in the adolescent

Can present with either primary or secondary amenorrhea or in patients with severe oligomenorrhea (> 90 day cycles)

DIFFERENTIAL DIAGNOSIS

Gonadal dysgenesis:

- Turner syndrome 45,XO – most common

  Adolescents will present with delayed puberty

  Ovarian failure is due to accelerated atresia of the ovarian follicles

- Turner mosaic pattern
- 46,XY gonadal dysgenesis
- 46,XX gonadal dysgenesis

Radiation/chemotherapy exposure:

- Effect of radiation: age- and dose-related
- Prepubertal ovary less sensitive to damage
- Chemotherapeutic agents toxic to ovary especially alkylating agents (See Oncology patients and gynecologic issues, Chapter 36)

Autoimmune disorders:

- Associated with antibodies to other organs

    Adrenal, thyroid, parathyroid, pituitary

- Associated with other autoimmune states

    Myasthenia gravis, diabetes, pernicious anemia, vitiligo

Idiopathic cause

Rare causes:

- 17-hydroxylase deficiency
- Resistant ovary syndrome
- Galactosemia
- Myotonic dystrophy
- Trisomy 21
- Sarcoidosis
- Ataxia telangiectasia
- Mumps
- Tuberculosis
- Hemorrhagic ovary

DIAGNOSIS

Physical findings

Findings variable and dependent on whether the gonads have had some function

May see variable breast development and the presence of pubic hair

Laboratory tests

FSH level

- Should be repeated if elevated with no explanation (e.g., previous chemotherapy)

Karyotype

- Should be done if elevated FSH with no explanation
- If Y-chromosome present, remove gonads to prevent malignant transformation

If normal karyotype

- Check thyroid stimulating hormone, thyroxine, complete blood count, calcium, phosphorus, 8 a.m. cortisol
- Consider antibody titers to thyroid, adrenal, ovary, islet, parietal cells to rule out further autoimmune disorders

MANAGEMENT

Pediatric endocrinology consult may be helpful

Use estrogen and progestin medication to complete maturation of secondary sexual characteristics:

- Conjugated equine estrogen (CEE) 0.3 mg po every other day × 3 months
- Then advance to 0.3 mg CEE po per day × 3 months
- Then advance to 0.3 mg CEE po alternate with 0.625 mg po × 3 months
- Then advance to 0.625 mg CEE po × 3 months
- When spontaneous bleeding occurs or if no bleeding occurs by this time:

    Add medroxyprogesterone acetate 10 mg po days 16–25 of month to cycle patient

- After estrogen priming as above, can alternately use low-dose oral contraceptive pills

Consider baseline bone density evaluation with repeat in one year (see Osteoporosis, Chapter 38):

- Adolescents are accruing peak bone mineral density in puberty; any interruption as with POF can have a negative impact which should be documented, monitored and addressed

Patient and family members will need counseling due to the stress and long-term fertility ramifications of POF

PROGNOSIS

Hormone therapy can complete secondary sexual characteristics and maintain bone mineral density

Patients with POF may still be able to conceive; rare spontaneous ovulation has been reported

Successful use of donor oocytes has been reported to result in pregnancy in the POF patient

BIBLIOGRAPHY

Emans SJ. Delayed puberty and menstrual irregularities. In Emans SJ, Laufer MR, Goldstein DP, eds. *Pediatric and Adolescent Gynecology*, 4th edn. Philadelphia: Lippincott-Raven, 1998:163–262

Speroff L, Glass RH, Kase NG. *Clinical Gynecologic Endocrinology*, 6th edn. Baltimore: Lippincott Williams and Wilkins, 1999:430–48

48 Premenstrual dysphoric disorder (PMDD)

PMDD is the most severe form of premenstrual syndrome (PMS) with predominance of anger, irritability and internal tension

Present in 2–3% of women overall and in 1 of 6 women with PMS

Controversy whether exists in adolescents

DEFINITION

Distinct changes that occur during the last week of the luteal phase including markedly depressed mood, anxiety, affective lability, and anhedonia, with these symptoms being absent in the week after menses

Confirmation requires at least 2 prospectively charted cycles (using diaries) that correlate periodicity with symptoms *and* presence of 5 of the 11 specific symptoms (see below) *and* clear documentation of impairment

Need to investigate for comorbidity (major depression, bipolar and panic disorder) before concluding PMDD is sole diagnosis for presenting symptoms

DSM-IV criteria for PMDD:

Prospective documentation of physical/behavioral symptoms for most of preceeding year

Five or more of the following symptoms present during the week before menses, resolving within first few days after menses starts

At least one of the five symptoms must be one of the first four on list:

(1) Feeling sad, hopeless or self-deprecating

(2) Feeling tense, anxious, or 'on edge'

(3) Marked lability of mood interspersed with frequent tearfulness

(4) Persistent irritability, anger, and increased interpersonal conflicts

(5) Decreased interest in usual activities, which may be associated with withdrawal from social relationships

(6) Difficulty concentrating

(7) Feeling fatigued, lethargic, or lacking in energy

(8) Marked changes in appetite, which may be associated with binge eating or craving certain foods

(9) Hypersomnia or insomnia

(10) A subjective feeling of being overwhelmed or out of control

(11) Other physical symptoms, such as breast tenderness or swelling, headaches, joint or muscle pain, a sensation of bloating, weight gain

EVALUATION

Must differentiate PMDD from premenstrual exacerbation of an underlying major psychiatric disorder as well as medical conditions such as hyper- and hypothyroidism

History

Ensure regularity of menstrual cycles

IF cycles irregular (< 25 days or > 36 days):

- Perform appropriate endocrine evaluation (see Dysfunctional uterine bleeding, Chapter 13)

Obtain confidential sexual history

Physical examination

Assess for medical conditions

Evaluate for signs/symptoms of thyroid disease

Hypothyroidism: dry skin, goiter, delayed deep tender reflex, constipation, hair loss

Hyperthyroidism: tachycardia, tremors, exophthalmos, diarrhea, vomiting

Laboratory tests

Complete blood count, chemistry profile, thyroid stimulating hormone

MANAGEMENT

IF no medical condition identified:

Have patient record symptoms prospectively for 2 months with the Calendar of Premenstrual Experiences (COPE) (see Premenstrual syndrome, Chapter 49)

IF no documented symptom free interval in follicular phase:

Have patient evaluated for mood or anxiety disorder

IF documented symptom-free follicular phase:

Qualify for treatment as below

- (IF patient sexually active prescribe oral contraceptives in addition to treatment below)

Treatment

Selective serotonin reuptake inhibitors (SSRIs)

Fluoxetine (Serafem® or Prozac®)

- 20 mg po dose daily (FDA approved dose for PMS)
- 15% of patients will experience side-effects:

  Most common: Headache

  Nausea

  Anxiety/jitteriness
- 15% will not respond
- There is no evidence that increasing dose will improve response

Sertraline (Zoloft®)

- May be effective
- 50 to 150 mg/day throughout menstrual cycle

Non-responders:

Gonadotropin releasing hormone (GnRH) agonists

- Lupron Depot® 3.75 mg IM monthly
- Counsel patient/parent about potential bone loss
- Obtain pre- and post-treatment bone densitometry study (see Osteoporosis, Chapter 38)
- Give Aygestin® 5 mg po daily
- Instruct patient to have 1500 mg calcium intake daily (diet plus appropriate supplement) with 400 IU Vitamin D
- Encourage weight-bearing exercise

Alprazolam

- 0.25 mg tid or qid in luteal phase

    There is no literature on this in adolescents and this should be used only with a second opinion and great caution due to the addictive nature of the medication

BIBLIOGRAPHY

American Psychiatric Association. DSM-IV. *Diagnostic and Statistical Manual of Mental Disorders*, 4th edn., Washington DC: American Psychiatric Association, 1994

Bashford R, Horrigan JP. Progesterone organogel for premenstrual dysphoric disorder (Letter to the editor). *J Am Acad Child Adolesc Psychiatry* 2000;39:546–7

Mortola JF, Girton L, Beck L, *et al*. Diagnosis of premenstrual syndrome by a simple, prospective and reliable instrument: the Calendar of Premenstrual Experiences. *Obstet Gynecol* 1990;76:302

Van Leusden HA. Premenstrual syndrome no progesterone; premenstrual dysphoric disorder no serotonin deficiency. *Lancet* 1995;346:1443–4

49 Premenstrual syndrome

Recurrent severe physical, psychological and/or behavioral changes that result in interference with interpersonal relationships and normal activities and that occur in a cyclic fashion beginning 1 to 2 weeks prior to menses and resolve by the end of menstruation

Establish cyclic occurrence with prospective recording of symptoms on a calendar for 2–3 cycles. Have the patient list three to five symptoms that are the most concerning to her and track them daily. Review the symptom diary in 2 to 3 months

Calendar of Premenstrual Experiences (COPE) score of > 42 in luteal phase (see Figure 49-1)

PMS symptoms

Abdominal bloating – most common physical manifestation (90%)

Fatigue – most common behavioral symptom (90%)

PMS subjects can be identified based on the presence of at least one behavioral symptom and one physical symptom:

Behavioral	*Physical*
Fatigue	Abdominal bloating
Irritability	Breast tenderness
Depression	Headache
Expressed anger	Swollen extremities
Poor concentration	
Social withdrawal	

Name

Day of cycle	1	2	3	4	5	6	7	8	9	10	11	12	13	14	15	16	17	18	19	20	21	22	23	24	25	26	27	28	29	30	31	32	33	34	35	36
Date																																				
Menses																																				
BEHAVIORAL																																				
Fatigue																																				
Irritability																																				
Depression																																				
Expressed anger																																				
Poor Concentration																																				
Social withdrawal																																				
PHYSICAL																																				
Abdominal bloating																																				
Breast tenderness																																				
Headache																																				
Swollen extremities																																				
Acne																																				
Increased appetite																																				
GI symptoms																																				
Hot flashes																																				
Heart palpitations																																				
Dizziness																																				

Scale:

No symptom	0
Mild	1
Moderate	2
Severe	3
Menstrual flow	M

Therapy

Figure 49-1 Calendar of premenstrual experiences (COPE)

History

Menstrual history (menarche, cycle interval, length of flow)

Associated menstrual symptoms:

- Dysmenorrhea
- Nausea/vomiting/diarrhea

Onset of time with PMS symptoms and previous attempts at treatment

Impact of PMS symptoms on activities

- Missed school/activities

Past medical history:

Any past/chronic illnesses

Psychiatric disorders

Increased life stressors: change in school/divorce/death

Athletic endeavors

Physical examination

While typically the exam is normal, look for any organic cause of symptoms:

- Thyroid disorder
- Chronic diseases
- Pelvic pain due to ovarian cyst, endometriosis

Laboratory tests

Complete blood count (CBC), erythrocyte sedimentation rate (ESR) evaluate for anemia, chronic disease

Thyroid function tests (TFTs) – evaluate thyroid status

Other tests as indicated by exam (e.g. prolactin for galactorrhea)

TREATMENT

Non-pharmacologic treatments:

Assist patient with sense of control over PMS:

- Educate about disorder
- Encourage healthy diet/regular exercise

- Identify stressors/refer for help with stress reduction
- Reassess in 2–3 cycles

Medications:

If non-pharmacologic treatment is unsuccessful, start with the medications with lowest side effect profiles and established benefit from randomized control trials non-steroidal antiinflammatory drugs (NSAIDs) diuretics/selective serotorin reuptake inhibitors (SSRIs)

Start with NSAIDS, oral contraceptive pills (OCPs) or spironolactone. If no, success in 3 cycles then try SSRIs. In severe cases, consider short-term use of gonadotropin releasing hormone (GnRH) with add-back hormonal therapy, understanding the unknown full negative potential effect on adolescent and long-term bone density. Would obtain second opinion from appropriate specialist regarding the patient's specific symptoms (i.e. gastroenterology for nausea, neurology for headaches, etc.)

NSAIDs:

Mefenamic acid

- 250 mg every 8 h starting on cycle day 16
- Increase to 500 mg cycle day 19

Diuretics:

- Alleviate breast tenderness/bloating/perceived weight gain
- Spironolactone
  100 mg po daily from cycle day 12 until first day menses

Oral contraceptives:

May help especially teens with premenstrual seizures

SSRIs:

Fluoxetine 20 mg per day continuously

- May increase does up to 60 mg/day if needed but may have increased side effects

GnRH agoinsts:

Depot leuprolide acetate 3.75 mg monthly

- Counsel patient/parent re: risk of osteoporosis with use as well as side effect profile
- Obtain pre- and post-treatment bone densitometry study to document effect on bone density
- Give Aygestin (ESI Lederle, Inc., Philadelphia, PA) 5 mg po daily
- Ensure calcium supplement plus diet is 1500 mg/day

- Give 400 IU Vitamin D po daily

- Encourage weight bearing exercise

- Treatment for more than 6 months carries a significant risk of osteoporosis and limits long-term usefulness (see Osteoporosis, Chapter 38)

BIBLIOGRAPHY

Laufer MR, Goldstein DP. Dysmenorrhea, pelvic pain and the premenstrual syndrome. In Emans SJ, Laufer MR, Goldstein DP, eds. *Pediatric and Adolescent Gynecology*, 4th edn. Philadelphia: Lippincott-Raven, 1998

Mortola JF, Girton L, Beck L, *et al*. Diagnosis of premenstrual syndrome by a simple, prospective and reliable instrument: the Calendar of Premenstrual Experieces. *Obstet Gynecol* 1990;76:302

Mortola JF, Girton L, Fisher U. Successful treatment of severe premenstrual syndrome by combined use of gonadotropin-relaeasing-hormone agoinst and estrogen progestin. *J Clin Endocrinol Metab* 1991;72:A252–F252

Vellacott ID, Shroff NE, Pearce MY, *et al*. A double blind, placebo-controlled evaluation of spironolactone in the premenstrual syndrome. *Curr Med Res Opin* 1987;10:450

Wyatt D. Premenstrual syndrome. In *Clinical Evidence Concise*. London: BMJ Publishing Group, 2002

50 Prolactin disorders

Prolactin disorders may present with absent or abnormal menses and/or galactorrhea

May also present with delayed/arrested puberty, visual changes or headaches

CLINICAL EVALUATION

Physical examination

Visual field examination by direct confrontation

> If unclear, refer to ophthalmologist

Palpate thyroid for enlargement

Breast examination

> May need to compress the breast and squeeze nipple to demonstrate galactorrhea

Laboratory studies

Obtain a thyroid stimulating hormone (TSH) and a fasting prolactin level

Treatment

Based on specific cause of hyper- or hypoprolactinemia

Treatment may be lifelong

Can assess adequacy of treatment with yearly prolactin levels

HYPERPROLACTINEMIA

DEFINITION

Levels > the upper limit of assay (e.g. > 20–30 ng/ml)

DIFFERENTIAL DIAGNOSIS

Idiopathic

Post-partum/post-abortal state

Pituitary adenoma

Hypothyroidism

Hypothalamic disease/tumors:

- Craniopharyngioma
- Sarcoidosis
- Histiocytosis X
- Encephalitis
- Pituitary stalk compression

Pharmacological agents:

- Phenothiazines
- Reserpine
- Prostaglandins
- Methlydopa
- Amitriptyline
- Cimetidine
- Benzodiazepine
- Haloperidol
- Cocaine
- Metoclopromide

Chronic renal failure

Local causes:

- Chest wall surgery
- Trauma
- Nipple stimulation
- Herpes zoster
- Atopic dermatitis
- Thoracic burns

Normal variations:

- Lowest levels after fasting between 9 and 11 a.m.
- Increased levels after eating, coitus, stress, exercise

DIAGNOSIS

Prolactin > 20 but < 100 ng/ml

Repeat fasting level

Prolactin > 100 ng/ml

Order MRI to rule out pituitary abnormality/tumor

TREATMENT

Treat on basis of etiology of hyperprolactinemia

Dopamine agonists can be used both to suppress pituitary adenomas and to treat symptomatic galactorrhea

Treatment of idiopathic hyperprolactinemia

Use of dopamine agonists

Consult with pediatric endocrinologist before use

Bromocriptine (Parlodel®)

Start at bedtime to avoid initial postural hypotension

Use half of 2.5 mg tablet (1.25 mg initial dose)

Advance dose slowly, changing doses every 2–4 weeks after checking fasting prolactin level

Recommended dose advancement:

- 1.25 mg at bedtime
- 2.5 mg at bedtime
- 1.25 mg in the morning
- 2.5 mg at bedtime
- 2.5 mg in the morning
- 3.75 mg at bedtime

Side effects: Nausea, gastrointestinal upset

Can avoid these by placing oral tablet in the vagina for vaginal absorption

Cabergoline (Dostinex®)

0.5 mg tablet twice weekly, advance to 1.0 mg tablet

More expensive than bromocriptine

Better tolerated than bromocriptine

Treatment of hypothyroidism

Consult with pediatric endocrinology

Treat underlying disorder of hypothyroidism with thyroid replacement and hyperprolactinemia will resolve

Pituitary adenoma

Based on size

Undetectable by MRI:	Dopamine agonist
Microadenoma < 10 mm:	Dopamine agonist
Macroadenoma > 10 mm:	Dopamine agonist
	May offer surgical option/consult neurosurgeon

Treatment of hyperprolactinemia due to other pharmacologic agents

Medications causing hyperprolactinemia include:

Dopamine antagonists

Anti-psychotics

Once prolactin level obtained and there is documented absence of pituitary adenoma, treat symptomatic galactorrhea with dopamine agonists

Treatment of hyperprolactinemia associated amenorrhea

Successful medical treatment of hyperprolactinemia typically results in resumption of normal menses

Oral contraceptives may be indicated for those who remain amenorrheic dispite normal prolactin levels and for those sexually active teenagers with hyperprolactinemia regardless of treatment

Follow-up care

Follow patients with yearly prolactin levels

Levels typically remain between 30–100 mg

After 1 or 2 years suppression, may discontinue medicines with close follow-up

If levels increase, reevaluate with MRI as levels indicate and reinstitute dopamine agonist treatment

HYPOPROLACTINEMIA

DEFINITION

Levels less than the lower limit of assay (e.g. < 2 ng/ml)

DIFFERENTIAL DIAGNOSIS

Pituitary macroadenoma:

Large tumor may destroy pituitary lactotroph cells

Empty sella syndrome:

Congenital incompleteness of the sella turcica

- Diaphragm allowing fluid into space and separation/flattening of the pituitary
- Post-surgical

Post-radiation

Post-infarction of a pituitary tumor

Pseudohypoparathyroidism

TREATMENT

Macroadenoma destroying lactotroph cells:

Neurosurgical consult for evaluation and removal

Empty sella syndrome:

Follow with yearly prolactin levels

Consider annual coned-down radiographic imaging

BIBLIOGRAPHY

Emans SJ. Delayed puberty and menstrual irregularities. In Emans SJ, Laufer MR, Goldstein DP, eds. *Pediatric and Adolescent Gynecology*, 4th edn. Philadelphia: Lippincott-Raven, 1998:163–262

Katz E, Schran HF, Adashi EY. Successful treatment of a prolactin-producing pituitary macroadenoma with intravaginal bromocriptine mesylate: a novel approach to intolerance of oral therapy. *Obstet Gynecol* 1989;73:517–20

Soto-Albors CE, Randolph JF, Ying YK, *et al*. Medical management of hyperprolactinemia: A lower dose of bromocriptine may be effective. *Fertil Steril* 1987;48:213–17

51 Puberty

NORMAL PUBERTAL DEVELOPMENT

Usually between ages 8 and 13

	Mean age
Growth spurt:	9.6 years (peak height velocity 2.5 years later)
Thelarche	10.9 years
Pubarche	11.2 years
Menarche	12.7 years

DELAYED PUBERTAL DEVELOPMENT

DEFINITION

Absence of pubertal development by age 13 *or*

Delay in menarche with some pubertal development

Menses typically occur within 2–3 years of secondary sexual characteristic development so a halt in maturation should prompt an evaluation

DIFFERENTIAL DIAGNOSIS

Can be classified based on gonadotropin levels (follicle stimulating hormone levels (FSH))

Hypergonadotropic hypogonadism

[Increased FSH levels indicate ovarian failure]

Ovarian failure (See Premature ovarian failure, Chapter 47)

- Abnormal karyotype

    45,XO most common

- Normal karyotype

    46,XX

    46,XY

    galactosemia

    chemotherapy/radiation damage

    autoimmune disorders

Hypogonadotropic hypogonadism

[Low FSH indicates absent to low stimulation of the ovary]

Reversible causes

   Constitutional, physiologic delay – most common

   Central suppression (e.g. weight loss, anorexia, chronic diseases)

   Primary hypothyroidism

   Congenital adrenal hyperplasia (CAH)

   Prolactinoma

Irreversible causes

   GnRH deficiency (Kallman's syndrome) – most common

   Hypopituitarism

   Congenital central nervous system (CNS) lesion

   Other pituitary adenomas

   Craniopharyngioma

   Malignant pituitary tumor

Eugonadism

[Normal FSH levels with anatomic defect and some pubertal changes]

   Mullerian agenesis – most common

   Vaginal septum

   Imperforate hymen

   Androgen insensitivity

   Inappropriate positive feedback

EVALUATION

History

Age of initiation of pubertal development, if any, and rate of development

Neonatal history:

- Birth weight (Turner syndrome patients may be IUGR)
- Lymphedema (associated with Turner syndrome)
- Congenital anomalies (may also have uterovaginal anomaly)

Review of systems:

- Assess for items that would cause central nervous system suppression:

    Neurologic symptoms

    Inability to smell

    Weight changes/eating disorders

    Competitive athletics

    Chronic disease (e.g. Crohn's)

- Assess for symptoms indicative of vaginal septum/imperforate hymen

    Abdominal pain or mass

Past medical/surgical history:

- Chronic disease
- Previous surgery
- Chemotherapy/irradiation

Family history:

- Familial disorders include: delayed menarche, androgen insensitivity, CAH, some forms of gonadal dysgenesis
- Age of menarche of sisters, mothers, grandmothers, aunts
- History of ovarian tumors (e.g. gonadoblastomas)
- History of endocrine (autoimmune) disorders like thyroiditis

Physical examination

Check height/weight/plot on curves and compare with previous available data

General assessment for midline facial defects

- (may indicate hypothalamic–pituitary dysfunction)

Assess for stigmata of Turner syndrome

- (webbed neck, wide-spaced nipple, short stature)

Thyroid assessment for enlargement

Breast exam

- Tanner stage (Sexual Maturity Rating [SMR] breast)
- Assess breast for galactorrhea

External genitalia

- SMR or Tanner stage pubic hair
- Ensure patent hymenal opening
- Assess estrogen stimulation to hymen

    Estrogen causes thickening of the hymenal tissue vs the red thin tissue of an unestrogenized hymen

- Rectal exam

    Rule out pelvic mass/obstructed outflow tract

    Determine presence of a uterus

Imaging

Pelvic ultrasonography:

- To confirm uterine agenesis, mullerian anomalies or adnexal masses
  or
- To assess adolescents in whom a rectoabdominal/vaginal abdominal exam is not possible
- NOTE: Interpret ultrasound results with caution as unestrogenized uterus/ovaries may not be well visualized on ultrasound and may be incorrectly assumed to be absent

MRI:

- Consider if ultrasound is equivocal

Bone age:

- May help to assist with diagnosis:

    Menarche is linked closer to bone age than chronologic age

    Hypothyroidism tends to delay bone age

    In constitutional delay bone age is delayed

- May help to estimate final height in patients with pubertal delay

Laboratory tests

FSH

- Determine central or gonadal disorder

- High levels:

  Indicate gonadal failure, unless expected because of prior chemotherapy/radiation, repeat to confirm

  If persistently > 30 MIU/ml, order a karyotype to rule out gonadal dysgenesis

- Low to normal levels:

  Indicate central nervous system cause (e.g. stress, eating disorder)

Thyroid stimulating hormone, prolactin levels

DIAGNOSIS AND TREATMENT

Treat underlying cause:

- High FSH and 45,X karyotype or mosaic (e.g. 46,XX/45,X):

  Turner syndrome (see Turner syndrome, Chapter 60)

- High FSH and normal karyotype:

  Premature ovarian failure

  Evaluate and treat as premature ovarian failure (see Premature ovarian failure, Chapter 47)

  Will need hormone replacement (see Turner syndrome for regimen)

- High FSH and 46,XY karyotype:

  Swyer's syndrome (streak gonads with normal mullerian structures and lack of sexual development)

  Need hormone replacement (see Turner syndrome for regimen)

  Need surgical extirpation of gonadal streak

- Low to normal FSH:

  Exclude systemic disease, poor nutrition and treat accordingly

  If no systemic disease or eating disorder

  Consider MRI to rule out CNS defect or disorder

  Consider pediatric endocrinology consult

  May perform GnRH stimulation test to assess pituitary response

PRECOCIOUS PUBERTY

DEFINITION

Appearance of breast or pubic hair development before age 8 years

KEY POINTS

Precocious puberty may result in short stature due to premature closure of epiphyseal growth centers

Most cases of precocity are secondary to idiopathic premature maturation of the hypothalamic–pituitary–ovarian (HPO) axis with GnRH release

CLASSIFICATION OF CAUSES

Can be determined by answering the following questions:

Is the development due to a GnRH dependent or centrally active cause (premature activation of HPO axis with pituitary release of LH/FSH) or a GnRH independent or peripheral source (non-GnRH source) of stimulation (e.g. ovarian estrogen production)?

- GnRH dependant puberty (also called true, central or complete precocious puberty):

    Due to premature maturation of the HPO axis

    Pulsatile GnRH release stimulated pituitary release of FSH/LH

    Pituitary FSH/LH then stimulate ovarian estrogen production and eventual ovulation

- GnRH independant puberty (also called pseudoprecocious, peripheral or incomplete precocious puberty):

    Due to gonadotropin and sex steroid secretion occurring independently of hypothalamic GnRH stimulation of pituitary

Is the development isosexual or heterosexual (contrasexual)?

- Is the development consistent with the sex of the child?
- If so, then is isosexual
- If signs of virilization present, then development is heterosexual
- [See Contrasexual pubertal development, below]

Is this a non-progressive subclass of precocious puberty?

- Some changes may be isolated to either premature adrenal function (premature adrenarche) or breast development (premature thelarche)
- (See Premature thelarche, Premature menarche, Premature adrenarche, below)

DIFFERENTIAL DIAGNOSIS

GnRH dependent or true (central) precocious puberty

Idiopathic activation of HPO axis – most common (50–85% cases of precocity)

Cerebral disorders (7% cases of precocity):

- Congenital malformations – e.g. hamartomas
- Brain tumors – e.g. gliomas
- Brain abscess
- Hydrocephalus
- Infiltrative lesion
- Sequelae of cellular damage–radiation or infection
- Neurofibromatosis

GnRH independent or pseudo (peripheral) precocious puberty

Gonadal causes:

- Ovarian tumors (e.g. granulosa cell tumors, dysgerminomas)
- McCune–Albright syndrome
  - Syndrome of precocity/café-au-lait spots/cystic bone lesions

Adrenal causes

- Adrenal secreting tumors/CAH

Ectopic causes

- Human chorionic gonadotropin (hCG) secreting tumors

Exogenous causes

- Iatrogenic hormones (e.g. conjugated estrogens)

Hypothyroidism

- VanWyk syndrome
  - Precocity, hypothyroidism, hyperprolactinemia

NOTE: Prolonged or repeated exposure to estrogen from non-GnRH dependent causes may lead to central precocious puberty creating a crossover between central and peripheral causes

EVALUATION

History

What is the time course of changes?

- A normal tempo (breast then pubic hair) – more likely central cause
- Abrupt and rapid tempo – more likely estrogen sectreting lesion

Assess CNS symptoms or damage:

- History of birth trauma, encephalitis, seizures
- History of headaches, visual changes, nausea

Assess abdominal pain, urinary or bowel symptoms

Family history:

- Early puberty or unusual short stature
- Neurofibromatosis

Medications:

- Possible ingestion of exogenous estrogens

Physical examination

Height, weight and plot on growth curves

- Look for change in height velocity (i.e. patient was at 5% now at 50th% for height)

Perform gross visual field evaluation

Visualize optic discs

- Look for papilledema (i.e. signs and intercranial pressure with CNS tumor)

Examine skin for:

- Acne, apocrine odor, café-au-lait spots, hirsutism

Palpate thyroid:

- Hypothyroidism associated with thyromegaly, slow pulse, delayed relaxation phase of deep tendon reflexes

Evaluate breasts:

- Tanner stage, measure horizontal and vertical dimension
- Check for galactorrhea

Abdomen:

- Check for hepatosplenomegaly
- Check for masses

External genitalia:

- Tanner stage pubic hair
- Evaluate presence of estrogenization

  Pink, thickened hymen with mucus discharge indicates exposure to estrogen vs red, thin hymen of unestrogenized state

- Evaluate for clitoromegaly (glans > 5 mm)
- Rectoabdominal exam

  To check for ovarian enlargement/adnexal masses

Diagnostic tests

Basic laboratory:

- LH, FSH, estradiol levels
- TSH, hCG levels
- If virilized: check testosterone, dehydroepiandrosterone sulfate (DHEAS), and 7 a.m. hydroxyprogesterone acetate level

Bone age:

- A radiologic evaluation of non-dominant wrist
- Serial studies every 6 months can establish rate of skeletal maturation
- A bone age > 2 standard deviations than chronologic age is abnormal and unlikely to be a normal variant

Ultrasound of pelvis:

- Rule out pelvic mass

CT or MRI of CNS:

- Rule out CNS lesion

May need GnRH stimulation test:

- To evaluate pituitary response
- Administer 100 µg of GnRH IV
- Measure baseline and 20, 40, and 60 minute FSH/LH levels

  True (GnRH dependent) cases: see increase in LH > FSH

  Peripheral/non-GnRH cases: No increase in LH/FSH

If suspect McCune–Albright syndrome:

- Consult with pediatric endocrinologist
- Consider ordering a basal skull film or bone scan to look for lytic bone lesions

Table 51-1 Laboratory findings in disorders producing precocious puberty

	Gonadal size	Basal FSH/LH	Estradiol or testosterone	DHEAS	GnRH response
Idiopathic	Increased	Increased	Increased	Increased	Pubertal
Cerebral	Increased	Increased	Increased	Increased	Pubertal
Gonadal	Unilateral increase	Decreased	Increased	Increased	Flat
Albright	Increased	Decreased	Increased	Increased	Flat
Adrenal	Small	Decreased	Increased	Increased	Flat

From Speroff L, Glass RH, Kase NG. *Clinical Gynecologic Endocrinology and Infertility*, 5th edn. Baltimore: Williams & Wilkins, 1994:375. Used with permission from Turrentine JE, Aviles M, Novak JS (eds). *Clinical Protocols in Obstetrics and Gynecology*. New York: The Parthenon Publishing Group, 2000

Diagnosis based on laboratory findings

See Table 51-1

TREATMENT

Depends on cause, extent and progression of precocity and whether cause can be surgically removed

Consult with pediatric endocrinology

Treatment should be instituted when:

- Bone age is > 2 years more than that of chronologic age
- Girls with precocity less than 6 years of age
- Girls with menarche prior to age 8 years
- Progressive thelarche and pubarche leaving patient isolated/different from peers/psychologic/behavioral reasons

GnRH dependent causes:

- Treat with GnRH agonist

    Diminishes secretion of pituitary FSH/LH

    Not effective for non-central causes of precocity

    Leuprolide acetate (Lupron Depot®, TAP Pharmaceuticals, Lake Forest, IL) IM every 4 weeks

    Dosing: 7.5 mg (under 55 lbs)

    11.25 mg (55–85 lbs)

    15 mg (over 85 lbs)

Continue use until patient reaches mean age for stage of pubertal development (see Osteoporosis, Chapter 38)

After GnRH agonist discontinued:

Menarche occurs within 1–2 years

Pubertal changes proceed with normal pace

Eventual fertility is unimpaired

Non-GnRH or peripheral causes:

- Tumors:

    Extirpation

- Cysts:

    May regress if secondary to central etiology/hypothyroidism

    If centrally etiology treated/thyroid hormone replaced

    If associated with McCune–Albright block estrogen with testolactone therapy

- Hypothyroidism:

    Thyroid replacement

CONTRASEXUAL PUBERTAL DEVELOPMENT

DEFINITION

Precocious pubertal development with signs of virilization

Secondary to excess adrenal or ovarian androgens

PRESENTATION

Acne, hirsutism, and virilization

DIFFERENTIAL DIAGNOSIS

Congenital adrenal hyperplasia (CAH)

Cushing's syndrome with tumor-related androgen excess

Adrenal tumors

Androgen-secreting ovarian tumors

EVALUATION

History

When was onset of symptoms?

Any signs of abdominal mass?

>   Gastrointestinal changes, pain

Family history of CAH

Physical examination

Check skin for hirsutism, acne, apocrine odor, striae

Perform abdominal exam

>   Check for hepatosplenomegaly

>   Check for abdominopelvic masses

Examine external genitalia

>   Check for clitoromegaly

Perform rectoabdominal exam

>   Evaluate for pelvic masses

Laboratory tests

LH, FSH, estradiol

Testosterone, DHEAS level

Baseline (7 a.m.) 17-hydroxyprogesterone level (17-OHP)

Androstenedione

If all above normal, consider 24-hour urine cortisol collection

DIAGNOSIS

CAH (see Ambiguous genitalia, Chapter 1)

If 17-OHP > 100 ng/dl then do 1 hour ACTH stimulation test:

CAH patients will be > 300 ng/dl, likely > 1000 ng/dl

If 17-OHP > 300 ng/dl then CAH

Adrenal tumors:

DHEAS will be > 700 ng/dl

Perform CT/MRI of adrenals to further evaluate

Ovarian tumors:

Testosterone > 150 ng/dl

Need pelvic ultrasound to confirm

Cushing's syndrome:

Confirm with 24 hour urine cortisol collection

TREATMENT

Ovarian/adrenal tumors

Excise

Congenital adrenal hyperplasia

Glucocorticoid replacement

(see Ambiguous genitalia, Chapter 1)

If developed central precocity as a result of long standing CAH, may be a candidate for GnRH therapy

PREMATURE THELARCHE

DEFINITION

Unilateral or bilateral breast enlargement without other signs of sexual maturation

KEY POINTS

Probably a result of a transient increase in FSH or ovarian sensitivity to FSH

May eventually progress to full precocious puberty, therefore requires interval reevaluation

DIFFERENTIAL DIAGNOSIS

Idiopathic/self-limited

First sign of precocious puberty

McCune–Albright syndrome (see Precocious puberty, above)

PRESENTATION

May be asymmetric – one side 6–12 months before the other

Most commonly seen < 2 years of age

More common in very-low-birth-weight infants

Absent adrenarche

EVALUATION

History/physical examination

Check height/weight and plot on growth curves (see Obesity, Chapter 35)

Review medication/creams used by patient

Examine each breast:

   Tanner stage

   Measure dimension horizontal/vertical (12 to 6 o'clock; 9 to 3 o'clock)

Examine skin:

   Look for café-au-lait spots

Assess external genitalia:

   Look at the hymen for evidence of estrogenization

Imaging/laboratory tests

FSH, estradiol level

Bone age:

   Determine effect of estrogen on bone age

   If within 2 SD of chronologic age, not significant

   If > 2 years of chronologic age, workup as per precocious puberty

Consider pelvic ultrasound:

> Especially if bone age advanced

MANAGEMENT

If bone age normal, reassurance with careful follow-up

Most cases regress or stabilize with eventual age appropriate normal pubertal progression

Will need every 4–6 month follow-up as up to 18% develop central precocity

PREMATURE MENARCHE

DEFINITION

Isolated menses in absence of other signs of puberty

KEY POINTS

Premature menarche is a diagnosis of exclusion: first, must exclude other causes of prepubertal vaginal bleeding (see Vaginal bleeding in the prepubertal patient, Chapter 65)

True premature menarche is thought to be secondary to a similar pathophysiology to premature thelarche

DIFFERENTIAL DIAGNOSIS

Vaginal infection

> Group A beta-hemolytic streptococcus
>
> *Shigella*

Trauma

Vaginal foreign body

Vaginal tumors

McCune–Albright syndrome

EVALUATION

History

When does bleeding occur?

Is it cyclic in nature?

Is there any associated vaginal discharge or association with vaginal infection?

Has there been a history of vaginal/perineal trauma?

Physical examination

Height/weight and plot on growth curve

Evaluate for acceleration in growth

Assess skin for café-au-lait spots

Check breasts for development

Assess abdomen for masses

Assess external genitalia

Look for evidence of estrogenization/trauma/tumors

Look for vaginal discharge/foreign body

Obtain cultures for routine organisms and plate specifically for isolation of *Shigella*

After cultures obtained, consider irrigating vagina with saline via pediatric feeding tube to rule out foreign body

Conclude exam with rectal abdominal exam

- Rule out intravaginal foreign body via palpation of vagina thru rectum and assess pelvis for mass

MANAGEMENT

Treat as per etiology

If culture reveals bacterial cause – treat as per vaginitis (see Vulvovaginitis, Chapter 69)

If foreign body, remove if necessary under anesthesia

If tumor related, consult with pediatric surgery

If uncertain of diagnosis, consult with pediatric endocrinology

PREMATURE ADRENARCHE

DEFINITION

Isolated pubic and/or axillary hair before age 8 years

KEY POINTS

Thought to be due to early activation of adrenal androgen secretion

More common in children with darker pigment, neurological problems and obesity

Girls with premature adrenarche may be at increased risk for polycystic ovarian syndrome(PCOS)/and hyperandrogenism with insulin resistance

These patients will have normal bone ages (within 2 SD)

EVALUATION

Same assessment as contrasexual precocious puberty

Must rule out CAH, precocious puberty, adrenal or ovarian tumors

MANAGEMENT

If bone age normal, reassess patient in 3 to 6 months for progression of pubic hair and other secondary sexual characteristics

Pubertal development should be normal

Some will develop PCOS, therefore if no menses occurs 3 years after thelarche, reevaluate for PCOS

BIBLIOGRAPHY

Emans SJ. Delayed puberty and menstrual irregularities. In Emans SJ, Laufer MR, Goldstein DP, eds. *Pediatric and Adolescent Gynecology*, 4th edn. Philadelphia: Lippincott-Raven; 1998:163–262

Lebrothon MC, Bourguignon JP. Management of central isosexual precocity: diagnosis, treatment, outcome. *Opin Pediatr* 2000;12:394–9

52 Radiologic imaging for gynecologic conditions

ULTRASONOGRAPHY (US)

Key points

First line for diagnosis of benign abnormalities of the uterus, ovary, fallopian tube, cervix and kidney

No radiation risk

Types:

Gray scale transabdominal – most useful and widely used in evaluating female pelvic organs and kidneys

Gray scale transvaginal – use only in sexually active and the cooperative, older, tampon-using adolescent; helpful in diagnosing tuboovarian abscess (TOA) and pregnancy

Color Doppler – can help in diagnosis of ovarian torsion; absence of flow may reflect non-viability in conjunction with exam; presence of flow is non-specific

Transperineal (translabial) – useful in defining abnormalities of urethra, periurethral soft tissues, anterior rectum, distal gynecologic tract

MAGNETIC RESONANCE IMAGING (MRI)

Key points

Useful when ultrasound fails to well define congenital tract anomalies, especially mullerian duct and vaginal defects; vulvar masses

Specific views image specific organs:

T1-W views:

- Coronal: kidneys and ovaries
- Sagittal: uterus, vagina and spine

T2-W

- Sagittal: uterus and vagina
- Axial: ovaries, lower uterine segment, cervix, and vagina

Use of a special gelatin capsule inserted in the vagina can help determine the extent of a vaginal obstruction

May require sedation to allow child under the age of 7 years to keep still for length of procedure

COMPUTED TOMOGRAPHY (CT)

Key points

Valuable in major abdominal or pelvic trauma; pelvic or renal malignancies; postoperative complications, i.e. organ injuries, abscesses

Spiral views very helpful in ruling out appendicitis

Disadvantages:

Not helpful in routine screening of pelvic structures

Radiation dose is significant to the gonads

May require sedation to allow the child to keep still although not as long as MRI

Contrast is required in most cases, small risk of anaphylaxis and nephrotoxicity

GENITOGRAM

Key points

Valuable in defining anatomy in ambiguous genitalia and a single perineal opening

Procedure:

Place 5 or 8 Fr feeding tube in orifice

Inject Hypaque-cysto dye

Use fluoroscopy to image passage of dye and hence anatomy

Use in conjunction with cystogram and/or rectal contrast in selected cases

Disadvantages:

Uses radiation

Opening has to be large enough to place catheter

BIBLIOGRAPHY

Garel L, Dubois J, Grignon A, *et al.* US of the pediatric female pelvis: a clinical perspective. *Radiographics* 2001;21:1393–407

Lang IM, Babyn P, Oliver GD. MR imaging of paediatric uterovaginal anomalies. *Pediatr Radiol* 1999;29:163–70

Maudgil DD, McHugh K. Role of computed tomography in modern paediatric uroradiology. *Eur J Radiol* 2002;43:129–38

Teele RL, Share JC. Transperineal sonography in children. *Am J Radiol* 1996;168:1263–7

53 Rape

DEFINITIONS

Traditional: forced vaginal penetration of a woman by a male assailant; some states have made it gender neutral

Criminal sexual assault: any genital oral or anal penetration by a part of the accused's body or by an object, using force or without the victim's consent

Acquaintance rape: those sexual assaults committed by someone known to the victim, frequently a date, teacher, employer or family member

Incest: perpetrator is related to the victim by blood or by marriage

Statutory rape: sexual intercourse with a female under a specified age (varies by state)

Child sexual abuse: sexual assault occurring in childhood

IDENTIFICATION OF THE VICTIM

Key points

More than 75% of adolescent rapes are committed by an acquaintance of the victim; adolescent may fail to recognize behavior as violent

Use of substances: alcohol, marijuana, cocaine, benzodiazapines, and the date rape drugs (Rohypnol/flunitrazepam and gamma hydroxbutyrate) may cloud the person's consciousness or memory

Clinician's role

Assess patient for occurrence

Acute situation: medical and counseling services; inform victim of her rights and refer to legal assistance; help develop strategies to avoid future victimization

Remote situation: recognize behavioral and physical health signs suggestive of a previous sexual assault (see also Table 53-1):

Early initiation of voluntary sexual activity

Unintended pregnancy

Poor use of contraceptives

Involvement with significantly older man (defined as at least 5 years older)

At every routine screening visit despite the complaint, the adolescent should be queried regarding their past sexual experience with such questions as:

- Have you ever had sex?
- How old were you at your first sexual experience?
- Did you choose to have sex?
- Has anyone forced you to have sex?
- Has anyone ever touched you in a way that made you feel uncomfortable?
- Would you like to ask me any questions?
- **Record answers and non-verbal cues**

Intervention

Allow patient to describe the experience at a comfortable pace and in her own words; encourage expression of feelings

Be aware of the three stages of rape trauma syndrome

(1) trauma (fear of being alone, fear of men, sexual problems, depression)

(2) denial (not wanting to talk about it)

(3) resolution (dealing with fears and feelings and regaining a sense of control over life)

Counseling referral to mental health professional trained in the treatment of sexual assault should be offered initially and then periodically when significant future events (i.e. graduation, marriage, pregnancy) bring back the issue(s)

Comply with the legal requirements of the particular state as far as reporting; should be done in a sensitive manner and must preserve the safety of the adolescent victim

Prevention strategies:

Educate the patient:

You have the right to say no to sexual activity

You have the right to set sexual limits and insist that your partner honor them

Be assertive

Stay sober and watch out for dates or anyone else who tries to get you high

Never leave a party with someone you don't know well

Trust your feelings and intuitions. If it feels wrong it is

Communicate with and educate your friends and dates about sexual assault

No one should be raped or otherwise forced, coerced, or pressured into engaging in any unwanted sexual behavior

Physical examination and laboratory tests

If the last episode of the assault occurred less than 72 hours from presentation:

Careful examination often with photographic records

Collection of forensic evidence (see Sexual abuse, Chapter 54)

Collection of culture, wet prep and serology tests for sexually transmitted diseases (STDs) (see Sexual abuse, Chapter 54)

Pregnancy test – Quantitative human chorionic gonadotropin (hCG)

Repeat cultures, a wet prep, pregnancy test 1–2 weeks after the initial if prophylaxis was not given

Serologic tests for syphilis and HIV should be repeated 6 weeks after the initial if negative and assailant likely to be infected

May need to refer to emergency center if no capability locally

If the last episode of the assault more than 72 hours from presentation:

Collection of culture, wet prep and serology tests for STDs (see Sexual abuse, Chapter 54)

Pregnancy test – quantitative hCG

Depending on proximity of visit in relation to assault, may need to repeat certain tests to confirm they are truly negative; use guidelines in < 72 h section above

Prophylaxis (consider only if assault within 72 hours of presentation):

CDC 2002 recommends an empiric antimicrobial regimen for syphilis, *Chlamydia trachomatis, Neisseria gonorrhoeae*, trichomonas, bacterial vaginosis may be administered:

- Ceftriaxone 250 mg im in a single dose PLUS
- Metronidazole 2 g po in a single dose PLUS
- Azithromycin 1 g po in a single dose OR
- Doxycycline 100 mg po bid for 7 days

An emergency contraceptive regimen should be offered if pregnancy test is negative (**can be prescribed up to 120 h post-assault**) (see Emergency contraception, Chapter 16)

For both medication regimes the provider may want to consider anti-emetic medications

Hepatitis B vaccination without HBIG should adequately protect against hepatitis B virus if not previously vaccinated; follow-up doses should be administered 1–2 and 4–6 months after the first dose

For HIV prophylaxis:

> Review HIV/AIDS local epidemiology and assess risk for HIV infection in assailant
>
> Evaluate circumstances of assault that may affect risk for HIV transmission
>
> Consult with a specialist in HIV treatment if post-exposure is considered
>
> If the victim appears to be at risk for HIV transmission from the assault, discuss antiretroviral prophylaxis, including toxicity and unknown efficacy
>
> If the survivor chooses to receive antiretroviral post-exposure prophylaxis, provide enough medication to last until the next return visit; reevaluate survivor 3–7 days after initial assessment and assess tolerance of medications (see Sexual abuse, Chapter 54, for dosing)
>
> Perform HIV antibody test at original assessment; repeat at 6 weeks, 3 months, and 6 months

BIBLIOGRAPHY

Adolescent Victims of Sexual Assault. ACOG Educational Bulletin 1998 (252):1–5
Sexually Transmitted Diseases Treatment Guidelines 2002. *MMWR* 2002;51(RR-6)

Table 53-1   Behavioral and physical health signs suggestive of previous sexual assault

Behavioral and psychologic sequelae that may suggest a history of sexual assault

Teen pregnancy

Poor contraceptive use

Substance abuse (drug and alcohol)

Prostitution

Multiple sexual partners

Sexual dysfunction

Problems with interpersonal and sexual relations

Poor self-esteem

Depression/anxiety

Somatization

Eating disorders/obesity

Insomnia and nightmares

Suicidal attempts

Psychiatric admissions

Post-traumatic stress disorder

School failure

Physical health problems that may suggest a history of sexual assault

Chronic abdominal pain

Chronic pelvic pain

Gastrointestinal tract symptoms (irritable bowel syndrome and other gastrointestinal symptoms)

Vulvodynia and dyspareunia

Breast pain

Chronic gynecologic infections

Multiple STDs

Chronic headache

Musculoskeletal complaints

Multiple physical complaints

Reproduced with permission from American College of Obstetricians and Gynecologists. *Adolescent Victims of Sexual Assault.* Educational Bulletin, number 252, October 1998. © ACOG

54 Sexual abuse

Definition

Contact or interaction between a child and an adult when the child is being used for the sexual stimulation of the adult or another person

May also be committed by a minor either when that person is significantly older or in a position of power or control over that child

Diagnosis most commonly made by history as the physical exam is generally normal

Should be performed by an individual with significant experience in child sexual abuse assessment

Begins with interview of the caretaker, then if possible the child separately

> Non-direct and open-ended questions regarding: time, location, description of the scene, name and description of the perpetrator, and type of sexual acts

> 'What happened? Who did this? Where did it happen? When did it happen?'

> Use of anatomically correct dolls or play interviews may be helpful

> Level of response is age dependent (e.g. A 2-year old can answer who did something, an older child can tell you when)

> See Table 54-1 for a template of interview questions

If the healthcare provider has reasonable cause to suspect child abuse, a report to the state or local child-protection agency should be made

Clinical indicators

Behavioral signs and symptoms:

> Night terrors

> Changes in sleep habits

Clinging

Sexual acting out

Aggression

Regression

Eating disturbances

Physical complaints:

Recurrent somatic complaints of abdominal pain

Headaches

Vaginal pain

Dysuria

Encopresis

Enuresis

Hematochezia

EVALUATION

Physical examination

Urgency depends on how soon after the event the child presents for care

If the child presents within 72 hours of the last episode, forensic evidence should be collected

General physical examination:

Precedes the genital exam

Examine the skin and breasts for bruises or lacerations

Examine the oral cavity for bruising, petechiae, or lacerations

Examine the abdomen for tenderness or mass

Genitalia examination:

Should include inspection of the medial aspects of the thighs, labia majora and minora, clitoris, urethra, periurethral tissue, hymen, hymenal opening, fossa navicularis, posterior fourchette and anus

Photographic documentation of any visible trauma or lesions recommended

Use of a colposcope is helpful but not required to magnify and photograph at same time

Examination of the prepubertal girl's genitalia and anus both supine in frog-leg and prone in knee–chest position (See Gynecologic examination, pediatric patient, Chapter 21)

Table 54-1   Interviewing children about sexual abuse

I.   Initial procedure
    a.   A. Obtain information from parent, social worker or significant other without the child present
    b.   Ask child's terminology for genitalia

II.   Interview child alone in non-threatening environment (if possible, not in examination room)

III.   Establish rapport with child (play, color, ask child's name and age)
    a.   Ask about household
        1.   Where does child live?
        2.   With whom does child live?
        3.   Where does child sleep?
        4.   Does child go to school? Where?
    b.   Identify body parts (may want to use a diagram, or dolls – anatomically correct not necessary)
        1.   Identify all body parts – eyes, nose, hair, hands, belly button, as well as genitalia

IV.   Begin to focus on possibility of abuse
    a.   'Do you know why you came to see me?'
    b.   'Do you know what kind of doctor I am? I am a doctor who checks children's hearts, listens to their lungs, and also checks their private parts. Do you need your private parts checked?'
    c.   'Some children who come to see me tell me that someone has touched their private parts in a way that makes them feel uncomfortable. Has anything like that happened to you?'

V.   What happened?
    a.   Where were you?
    b.   Who was there?
    c.   Where was Mommy? Daddy?
    d.   Who did it?
    e.   What did he/she do?
    f.   Where were your clothes? Panties? His/her clothes?
    g.   When did it happen? One time/more than one time? Christmas time? After school? Dark/light outside?
    h.   Did you tell anyone? Who did you tell?

VI.   More specific questions (examples)
    a.   Establish the child's term for penis and identify on doll, drawing
    b.   What does he do with his penis?
    c.   What is it for?
    d.   What did you see it do?
    e.   What did the penis look like?
    f.   Did anything come out of it?
    g.   What was it like?
    h.   Where did it go?

(Continued)

VII. Concluding the interview?
   a. Thank patient for speaking with you
   b. Reassure child that they did a good job speaking with you and it was not his/her fault that something happened
   c. Tell the child that you believe what he/she said

VIII. Explain the examination
   a. 'Now we need to check you out – listen to your heart, lungs; feel your tummy; and look at your private parts'
   b. Describe how the pelvic exam will be performed/show patient the colposcope

IX. Don't
   a. Ask children leading question (e.g. Johnny touched you here, didn't he?)

X. Document
   a. Document questions asked and answers given
   b. Try to record exact words and phrases

XI. Modifications for adolescent
   a. Obtain more specific information: date and time of assault, history of assault (oral, rectal or vaginal penetration, oral contact by the offender, ejaculation (if known), digital penetration or penetration with foreign object)
   b. Obtain history of any self-cleaning activities (bathing, teeth brushing, urination, douching, changing clothes)
   c. Obtain menstrual history and whether patient uses contraception. Were any lubricants or a condom used?

Used with permission from Jacqueline M. Sugarman, MD. Evaluation of child sexual abuse. In Giardino AP, Darner EM, Asher JB. *Sexual Assault: Victimization Across the Life Span. A Clinical Guide.* St Louis: GW Publishing Inc., 1997;58

For menstruating girls with a history of vaginal penetration a full pelvic should be performed. Preparing the patient by showing them a video demonstrating the procedure can be helpful (see Bibliography)

Location of abnormalities should be described as on a clock face with the urethra in the 12 o'clock and anus in the 6 o'clock, respectively

Important to recognize that significant injuries to the perineum that result in lacerations can heal with little residua within a month of the assault

Suspicious physical findings for sexual abuse:

- Unexplained vulvar or vaginal erythema
- Unexplained vaginal discharge and/or bleeding
- See Hymenal anatomy, Chapter 25, for diagnostic hymenal findings
- Perianal findings:

   Fissures, tears and anal dilatation. Dilatation more than 20 mm without stool present is uncommon (1.2%) and suspicious

Table 54-2 Implications of commonly encountered sexually transmitted diseases (STDs) for the diagnosis and reporting of sexual abuse of infants and prepubertal children

STD confirmed	Sexual abuse	Suggested action
Gonorrhea*	Diagnostic⁺	Report‡
Syphilis*	Diagnostic	Report
HIV§	Diagnostic	Report
Chlamydia*	Diagnostic⁺	Report
Trichomonas vaginalis	Highly suspicious	Report
Condylomata acuminata* (anogenital warts)	Suspicious	Report
Herpes (genital location)	Suspicious	Report#
Bacterial vaginosis	Inconclusive	Medical follow-up

*If not perinatally acquired
⁺Use definitive diagnostic methods such as culture or DNA probes
‡To agency mandated in community to receive reports of suspected sexual abuse
§If not perinatally or transfusion acquired
#Unless there is a clear history of autoinoculation. Herpes 1 and 2 are difficult to differentiate by current techniques

Used with permission from Committee on Child Abuse and Neglect. American Academy of Pediatrics. Guidelines for the evaluation of sexual abuse of children: subject review. *Pediatrics* 1999;103:186–91. © 1999, AAP

Laboratory tests

Screen for *Neisseria gonorrhoeae* (GC) and *Chlamydia trachomatis* (CT) on culture media only and bacterial vaginosis (BV) and *Trichomonas* with wet prep within 72 hours of the last event or when it is known if penetration or ejaculation occurred or if there is discharge. In a menstruating female, obtain from cervix; in a prebubertal child from the deep vagina with a Dacron wire swab. GC also from anus and oropharynx; CT also from the anus

Screen for human papillomavirus (HPV) or herpes if wart or vesicular lesion present respectively

Serologic testing for syphilis, HIV and hepatitis B&C virus may be considered on an individual basis

Pregnancy test in a menstruating female

Implications of the diagnosis of a sexually transmitted disease (STD) for the reporting of child sexual abuse are outlined in Table 54-2

Forensic evaluation

Can obtain a 'rape kit' from your local child protective service, emergency ward, state police unit

Description of the specimens to be taken and how to obtain the specimens is listed in the kit

All persons handling the materials must sign for them to maintain the chain of evidence; if the kit needs to be stored in the clinician's office, it should be inaccessible and preferably in a locked area unit it can be given to the police or forensic laboratory

Specimens to be collected

General:

> Outer- and underclothing, if worn during or immediately following the assault
>
> Fingernail scrapings
>
> Dried and moist secretions and foreign material observed on the patient's body
>
> Wood lamp for detection of semen

Oral cavity:

> Swabs for semen (2) if within 6 hours of the assault
>
> Culture for *N. gonorrhoeae*
>
> Saliva for reference

Genital area:

> Dried and moist secretions and foreign material
>
> Combing of pubic hair, collection of all loose hair and foreign material
>
> Vaginal swabs (3)
>
> Wet-mount slide
>
> Dry-mount slides (2)
>
> Culture for *N. gonorrhoeae* and *C. trachomatis*

Anus:

> Dried and moist secretions and foreign material
>
> Rectal swabs (2)
>
> Dry-mount slides (2)
>
> Culture for *N. gonorrhoeae* and *C. trachomatis*

Blood:

> Blood type
>
> Test for syphilis

Test for pregnancy (or urine)

Alcohol/drug toxicology (or urine)

Urine:

Pregnancy (or blood)

Alcohol/drug toxicology (or blood)

Urinalysis with microscopy

Other:

Saliva – use sterile saline moistened clean gauze or filter paper to wipe area where saliva contamination present

Head hair

Pubic hair

MANAGEMENT

(1) Repair of injuries and treatment of venereal diseases

(2) Protection against further abuse

(3) Emotional support to the victim and her family

Repair of injuries

Most victims do not sustain serious physical injury as a result of the assault, particularly if they have been sexually active prior to the assault

See Genital trauma, Chapter 20, for specific recommendations

Treatment of sexually transmitted diseases (STDs)

Adolescent:

If within 72 hours of last act:

Emergency contraception (ECP), if pregnancy test negative (see Emergency contraception, Chapter 16)

Sexually transmitted disease prophylaxis (see Rape, Chapter 5)

HIV prophylaxis until results back (optional): (see Table 54-3)

Vaccination for hepatitis B (at baseline, 1–2 months and 4–6 months) if not given; without hepatitis B immune globulin (HBIG)

Follow-up serologic tests for syphilis and HIV should be repeated at 12 weeks after the assault if initial results were negative and these infections are likely to be present in the assailant

For ECP and STD medication regimes may want to provide antiemetic (See Emergency contraception, Chapter 16)

Follow-up pregnancy test if misses a period

Child:

If within 72 hours of last act:

Presumptive treatment is not recommended as prevalence of most STDs is low in prepubertal children

STD treatment: (see Sexually transmitted diseases, Chapter 56). Work with a pediatric pharmacist or infectious diseases specialist

HIV prophylaxis until results back (optional): (see Table 54-3)

Vaccination for hepatitis B (at baseline, 1–2 months and 4–6 months) if not given; without HBIG

Follow-up serologic tests for syphilis and HIV should be repeated at 12 weeks after the assault

Adolescent and child seen over 72 hours from last sexual act, await results; encourage vaccination for hepatitis B; ECP can be given up to 120 hours after assault

Counseling

Essential to optimal recovery for both victim and family

Referral sources:

Child advocacy center

Rape crisis center

Police agency

Sequelae can manifest in significant psychologic symptoms as an adult:

Sexual dysfunction

Drug addiction

Eating disorders

Promiscuity

Pelvic pain

Chronic vaginitis

Suicide ideation

Table 54.3 Dosage and administration of selected antiretroviral drugs that might be used for prophylaxis after exposure to HIV in children or adolescents

Drug generic name (abbreviation), trade name	Recommended dosage	How supplied
Nucleoside reverse transcriptase inhibitors (NRTIs)		
ZDV, Retrovir	Preterm infants (investigational)	Syrup: 10 mg/ml
	0–2 wk of age:1.5 mg/kg/dose, twice daily, orally (1.0 mg/kg/dose, every 12 h, IV)	Capsules: 100 mg
	> 2 wk of age: 2.0 mg/kg/dose, 3 times/day, orally (1.5 mg/kg/dose, every 8 h, IV)	Tablets: 300 mg
	Term infants	Combination (Combivir): ZDV, 300 mg, plus lamivudine, 150 mg, in a single tablet
	0–6 wk of age: 4 mg/kg/dose, twice daily, orally (3.0 mg/kg/dose, every 12 h, IV)	Injection: 10 mg/ml in 20-ml vials
	4 wk–12 y of age: 160 mg/m^2/dose, 3 times/day, orally, or 180–240 mg/ m^2/dose, twice daily, orally (maximum 200 mg/dose, 3 times/day or 300 mg/ dose, twice daily)	
	≥ 13 years of age: 200 mg/dose, 3 times/day, orally or 300 mg/dose, twice daily, orally	
ddI, Videx	< 3 mo of age: 50 mg/m^2/dose, twice daily, orally (investigational)	Chewable tablets*: 25 mg, 50 mg, 100 mg, 150 mg (2 tablets/dose)
	3 mo–12 y of age: 90–135 mg/m^2/dose, twice daily, orally or 240 mg/m^2/dose once daily, orally (investigational)	Buffered powder packets: mix with water: 100 mg, 167 mg, 250 mg
	13 y of age:	Coated tablets (Videx EC): 125 mg, 200 mg, 250 mg 400 mg
	< 60 kg in body weight: Tablets, 125 mg, twice daily, orally Powder, 167 mg, twice daily, orally	Pediatric powder for oral solution mixed to final concentration of 20 mg/ml or 10 mg/ml
	≥ 60 kg in body weight: Tablets, 200 mg, twice daily, orally, 400 mg, once daily, orally Powder, 250 mg, twice daily, orally, or 500 mg, once daily, orally	

(Continued)

Drug	Dose	Formulation
d4T, Zerit	<30 kg in body weight: 1 mg/kg/dose, twice daily, orally; 30–60 kg: 30 mg, twice daily, orally; >60 kg: 40 mg, twice daily, orally	Solution: 1 mg/ml; Capsules: 15, 20, 30, 40 mg. Mix with applesauce
3TC, Epivir	<1 mo of age: 2 mg/kg/dose, twice daily, orally; <37.5 kg in body weight: 4 mg/kg/dose, twice daily, orally; ≥37.5 kg in body weight: 150 mg/dose, twice daily, orally	Oral solution: 10 mg/ml; Tablets: 150 mg; Combination (Combivir): ZDC, 300 mg, plus 3TC, 150 mg, in a single tablet

Protease inhibitors (PIs)

Drug	Dose	Formulation
RTV, Norvir	3 mo–12 y of age: 400–450 mg/m^2/dose, twice daily, orally; 13 y of age: 600 mg/dose, twice daily, orally	Oral solution: 80 mg/ml; Gelcaps: 100 mg
IDV, Crixivan	3–12 y of age: 450 to 500 mg/m^2/dose, 3 times/day, orally; ≥13 y of age: 800 mg, 3 times/day, orally	Capsules: 200 and 400 mg. Must be stored in original bottle
NFV, Viracept	1 mo–12 y of age: 30–50 mg/kg/dose, 3 times/day, orally, or 55 mg/kg/dose, twice daily, orally (maximum 2000 mg/dose); ≥13 y of age: 750 to 1250 mg/dose, 3 times/day, orally, or 1250 mg/dose, twice daily, orally	Powder for oral suspension: 50 mg/'level scoop'
LPV/r, Kaletra	Children: LPV, 300 mg/m^2/dose, plus RTV, 75 mg/m^2/dose, twice daily, orally; Adults: LPV, 400 mg/dose, plus RTV, 100 mg/dose, twice daily, orally, or LPV, 533 mg/dose, plus RTV, 133 mg/dose, twice daily, orally if given with nevirapine	Oral solution: 400 mg of LPV/100 mg of RTV per 5 ml (80 mg of LPV/20 mg of RTV per ml). Can store at room temperature for 2 mo

ZDV, Zidovudine; IV, intravenous; ddI, didanosine; d4T, stavudine; 3TC, lamivudine; RTV, ritonavir; IDV, indinavir sulfate; NFV, nelfinavir mesylate; LPV/r, lopinavir/ritonavir. *Although the doses listed for adults are usually the Food and Drug Administration-licensed doses, the doses listed for children may be higher than the Food and Drug Administration-licensed doses. Before prescribing, see package insert for complete prescribing information, including drug toxicities, potential drug interactions, and contraindications for use. Used with permission of American Academy of Pediatrics from Havens PL, Committee on Pediatrics AIDS. Postexposure prophylaxis in children and adolescents for nonoccupational exposure to human immunodeficiency virus. Pediatrics 2003;111:1475–89

BIBLIOGRAPHY

Committee on Child Abuse and Neglect. American Academy of Pediatrics. Guidelines for the evaluation of sexual abuse of children: subject review. *Pediatrics* 1999;103:186–91

Havens PL, Committee on Pediatric AIDS. Post exposure prophylaxis in children and adolescents for nonoccupational exposure to human immunodeficiency virus. *Pediatrics* 2003;111:1475–89

Muram D. The medical evaluation in cases of child sexual abuse. *J Pediatr Adolesc Gynecol* 2001;14:55–64

Wilson B. *First Pelvic Exam Video.* Hollywood CA: Lange Productions

55 Sexual activity

Initiation of sexual intercourse during adolescence remains the norm for American youth

Among women ages 15–19 most pregnancies are unintended, and approximately 1 in 3 end in abortion

Overall rates of sexually transmitted diseases (STDs) in the United States are among the highest in the industrialized world

Children most likely to engage in earlier sexual activity include those:

> with learning problems or low academic attainment

> with other social, behavioral, or emotional problems (including mental health disorders and substance abuse)

> from low-income families

> from some ethnic minorities

> who are victims of physical and sexual abuse

> in families with marital discord and low levels of parental supervision

Many gay, lesbian, and bisexual youths can be at high risk:

> increased unsafe sexual practices with same or opposite sex partners

> increased rates of: depression, school drop out, homelessness and substance abuse

Rates of sexual activity with adolescents with disabilities are the same as those without; less likely to receive any sexuality education

HEALTHCARE PROVIDER

Key points

> Important role in discussions of adolescent health and sexuality

HEADS acronym to obtain social history (see High risk behaviors, Chapter 23, for more complete history profile)

- Home
- Education/employment
- Activities, ambition
- Drugs, diet, delinquency
- Sex, suicide

Certain principles in dealing with the adolescent

- Maintain confidentiality
- Reflect principles of normalization/acceptance
- Be respectful
- Avoid assumptions/judgments
- Specific questioning (see references below)
- Listen to responses
- Avoid medical jargon
- Recognize the links of other risk behaviors with sexual activity
- Think prevention
- Know your community resources for specific adolescent needs

Specific goals

- Delay initiation of sexual intercourse
- Encourage abstinence among sexually experienced youth
- Increasing the use of condoms and other forms of contraception

Sexuality history/counseling

Should be based on stages of adolescent development

All stages:

ACTION: Starting at Tanner 2 around the ages of 10–12, adolescent should initially and yearly fill out a confidential questionnaire (see Gynecologic examination, Chapter 21, Figure 21-14) and have time alone with the physician. After the introductions, the healthcare provider should outline the staging of the visit:

(1) History-taking with parent present

(2) Confidential (review the questionnaire and other risk issues) time alone with adolescent patient

(3) Physical exam with or without the parent

(4) Wrap-up with both parent and child

(5) If the parent claims: 'Oh we discuss everything' it is important to validate that. One can stop at this point or if there are significant issues brought out by the confidential questionnaire, one can pursue the time alone as standard but emphasizing that the young person can share with the parent everything discussed

(6) Good introductory references (see below) can lay the framework for future open communication

Early adolescence (ages 10–14):

Patients begin pubertal growth and development; begin to separate from parents and family; place an increased importance on same-sex peer relationships; are still concrete thinkers, have limited abilities to anticipate future consequences; are preoccupied with their own bodies, uncertain about their appearance; think a lot about the opposite sex, have crushes but rarely a relationship; inquire about issues such as masturbation

ACTION:

(1) Discuss with adolescent and parent about the sequence of pubertal physical changes

(2) Discuss with adolescent and parent about normalcy of same sex crushes, masturbation, homosexual experimentation and fantasies

(3) Discuss with the adolescent about alcohol and other substances

(4) Discuss with the adolescent about the dangers of oral sex

(5) ETR Associates has excellent teen based information materials appropriate to these topics and designed for the teen's educational level

Middle adolescence (ages 14–17):

Adolescents are at the end of their pubertal changes; display increased independence and conflict from their parents and are at the peak level of peer conformity; imagine the consequences but do not fully understand; common age when romantic relationships begin; romantic relationships typically monogamous but often short-lived; significant concerns about peer norms and begin to have questions about dating and fidelity

ACTION:

(1) Address self-esteem issues related to body image

(2) Support and praise for abstinence

(3) Address risk-taking behavior by reviewing the confidential questionnaire and asking what actions the teen would or is taking to avoid risk

(4) Discuss disease prevention in relation to specific risk behaviors

(5) ETR Associates has excellent teen based information materials appropriate to these topics and designed for the teen's educational level

Late adolescence (ages 17 and older):

Adolescents begin to take on a sense of responsibility for their health and have a more clearly defined body image and gender role; are more likely to conform to their parent's values rather than their peers; abstract thinking begins and enables them to understand others' thoughts and feelings; tend to engage in fewer risk behaviors as they can begin to conceptualize the consequences; emphasize supportive, intimate behaviors

ACTION: (If sexual debut earlier, should be addressed then)

(1) Discuss sexual dysfunction and sexual response

(2) Discuss relationships and mutuality

(3) Discuss methods to enhance compliance with contraception

(4) Explore support systems, partner attitudes and personal and parental expectations

PATIENT RESOURCES

Gravelle K, Gravelle J. *The Period Book*. New York: Walker and Company Publishing, 1996

Schaefer VL. *The Care and Keeping of You*. American Girl Library. Middleton, WI: Pleasant Company Publishing, 1998

ADOLESCENTS WITH DISABILITIES

Key points

Many parents seek contraception because they fear that the physical or intellectual limitations of their children make them at special risk for sexual assault

Provider needs to assess the social settings in which the youth is interacting with members of the same and opposite sex to determine if contraceptive prophylaxis is warranted

Sexual history needs to be taken as for any other young person (see above)

Disease or treatment may limit fertility and contraceptive methods (plans for treatment should be made in consultation with patient's medical specialist)

Sexual history/counseling

Discussions should be initiated with parents or guardians of children with disabilities at a young age to encourage self-protection and acceptable forms of sexual behavior

Provide sex education in an appropriate fashion: keep it simple, be repetitive, be aware of the particular condition's reproductive limitations, be aware of child's developmental level

Involve the patient with disabilities in their decisions about reproduction

Key issues in the contraceptive appropriateness are the intellectual functioning of the client, frequency of intercourse, and number of partners

Advocate the least permanent and intrusive method of contraception consistent with the lowest risk for the patient

Reversible contraception should be used whenever feasible (see Contraception, Chapter 11, for specific contraindications and cautions)

Sterilization should be the last option after all others have failed:

- Be familiar with the applicable law about sterilization of persons that are minors and/or have developmental disabilities in their particular jurisdiction
- Contact the particular state bar association using an Internet search directory such as:
  > Yahoo at dir.yahoo.com/government/law/organizations/ bar_associations and look for state bar of California at "http://www.calbar.org" or Massachusetts at "http://www.Massbar.org"
- Options for sterilization include tubal ligation or hysterectomy or tubal ligation with/without uterine ablation; choice depends on whether the goal includes pregnancy prevention or menstrual regulation or both

Many teens with certain medical disabilities are on potentially teratogenic medications and need to be aware of need for contraception:

Rheumatoid arthritis: gold salts; non-steroidal antiinflammatory drugs

Inflammatory bowel disease: 6-Mercaptopurine

Seizure disorders: Phenytoin, trimethadione, valproic acid

Cystic fibrosis: Sulfa drugs, tetracycline, ciprofloxacin

Cancer: Antimetabolites, alkylating agents, radiation

Inform adolescent patient/family of possible negative impact of disability on reproductive function

Inflammatory bowel disease: increased risk of infertility

Diabetes mellitus: increased risk of spontaneous abortion; dyspareunia associated with increased candida vulvovaginitis

Chemotherapy: decreased libido

Spinal cord injury: posttraumatic amenorrhea, loss of sensation

Cerebral palsy: spasms may cause vaginismus

Neurofibromatosis: increase in spontaneous abortion and stillbirth

Systemic lupus erythematosus: increased risk of prematurity and stillbirth

Chronic renal disease: increased risk of infertility

WEB SITE RESOURCES

www.ETR.org

www.aap.org

www.iwannaknow.org

www.naspag.org

www.nyacyuth.org (National Youth Advocacy Coalition)

www.seicus.org (Sex Information and Education Council of the United States)

www.teenshealth.org (Nermous Foundation)

BIBLIOGRAPHY

AAP Committee on Bioethics. Sterilization of minors with developmental disabilities. *Pediatrics* 1999;104:337–40

AAP Committee on Psychosocial Aspects of Child and Family Health and Committee on Adolescence. Sexuality education for children and adolescents. *Pediatrics* 2001;108:498–502

Blum RW. Sexual health contraceptive needs of adolescents with chronic conditions. *Arch Pediatr Adolesc Med* 1997;151:290–6

American College of Obstetricans and Gynecologists. *Tool Kit For Teen Care* 2003

Frankowski B. Sexual orientation of adolescent girls. *Curr Women's Health Rep* 2002;2:457–63

Garofalo R. Adolescent sexuality. *UpToDate* 2002;10(3)

Tobias BB, Ricer RE. Counseling adolescents about sexuality. *Primary Care; Clin Office Practice* 1998;25:49–70

56 Sexually transmitted diseases (STDs)

Rates of many STDs are highest in the adolescent population

> Chlamydia/gonorrhea rates are highest in females ages 15–19

The most common STD is human papillomavirus (HPV) infection

Younger teens (< 15 years) are at particular risk:

> More frequently have unprotected intercourse

> Are biologically more susceptible to infection

> Are engaged in partnerships of limited duration

> Face multiple obstacles in utilization of health care

In almost all states, adolescents in the US can consent for diagnosis and treatment of STDs without parental consent

Providers MUST remember to obtain an age appropriate confidential sexual history on all adolescents (see Gynecologic examination, Chapter 21 and High risk behaviors, Chapter 23)

Detailed treatment guidelines for STDs can be obtained at www.cdc.gov

CHLAMYDIA TRACHOMATIS

The highest rates for chlamydia are in adolescents and young adults

The majority of infections are asymptomatic and are only detected by screening

If left undiagnosed, 20–40% will result in pelvic inflammatory disease

Sexually active women should be screened at least annually and better still with each new sexual partner

Diagnosis

Pediatric cases:

> Culture: DNA probes or polymerase chain reaction (PCR) not approved in this patient population due to concerns about theoretic false positivies

Adolescent cases:

> Culture
>
> DNA probe
>
> PCR (urine or endocervical)

Management

Pediatric cases:

> Possible to have vertical transmission from mother to child/infant if diagnosed within 1st 3 years of life, but sexual abuse must be considered as possible etiology

Adolescent cases:

> Educate that short of abstinence, condom use for anal, vaginal and oral sex is the most effective way to prevent disease
>
> Stress need for routine screening includes screening with each new sexual partner and 4–6 weeks after treatment for chlamydia

Treatment

Children 45 kg:

> Erythromycin 50 mg/kg/day po divided into 4 doses daily for 14 days

Children > 45 kg but are < 8 years of age:

> Azithromycin 1 g orally in a single dose

Children > 8 years of age and adolescents:

> Azithromycin 1 g orally in single dose *or*
>
> Doxycycline 100 mg orally twice a day for 7 days
>
> (alternative therapies available at www.cdc.gov)

Follow-up

If patient infected, abstain from sexual intercourse for 7 days after azithromycin or until doxycycline regimen completed

Abstain from sex until partner treated

Most recent sexual partner should be referred for treatment as should any partner within prior 60 days.

Infected adolescents should be screened for reinfection 3 months after treatment for chlamydia

HEPATITIS A (HAV)

A viral infection transmitted by the fecal–oral route

Can be transmitted during sexual activity

Can be prevented with vaccination

Incubation period 28 days

Presentation

Can present as asymptomatic or symptomatic

Symptoms more common in adults

Asymptomatic more in children < 6 years

If symptomatic, happens suddenly

Fever, malaise, anorexia, nausea, abdominal pain within 15–45 days exposure

May progress to dark urine and jaundice

Symptoms usually resolve in 2 to 3 weeks

10–15% cases ill for up to 6 months

Diagnosis

Serologic testing: IgM antibody to HAV

Usually detectable 5 to 10 days before symptoms occur

Can be detected in serum for up to 6 months after infection

Management

Treatment

Supportive care

No dietary/activity restrictions

Hospitalization for dehydration associated with nausea/vomiting

Use medications metabolized by the liver with caution

Prevention

Vaccination

> For those at risk for sexual transmission

> For persons who use injection/non-injection illegal drugs

HEPATITIS B

A viral infection spread by blood and body fluids

Can be transmitted during oral, anal and vaginal sex

Incubation period of 60–90 days

1% of cases result in acute liver failure and death

One to 6 percent infected progress to carrier state or chronic infection that leads to liver failure and death

Can be prevented with vaccination

Presentation

Onset is gradual

Symptoms seen in only 30–50% patients > 5 years of age

Flu-like symptoms including anorexia, malaise, nausea, vomiting, abdominal pain, joint aches, fever

25% develop jaundice, dark urine and/or light stools 1–9 months after contracting the virus

Within 6 months, 90% patients recover with immunity to virus 6–10% adults, 25–50% children, and 70–90% infants develop chronic HBV – with 15–25% developing chronic liver disease

Transmission

Percutaneous (needle sticks, blood products, tattooing, etc.)

Permucosal (sexual intercourse, infected mother to infant)

Risk factors for infection

Multiple sexual partners (more than one partner in 6 months)

Recent history of an STD

Diagnosis

Serology

For acute hepatitis: HbsAg and anti-HBc IgM establish diagnosis

Then order HBV panel (see Table 56-1)

Management

Treatment

Acute infection: Supportive therapy

Chronic infection: Antiviral agents

Prevention

Hepatitis B vaccine

    When sexual abuse is identified, initiate vaccination in previously unvaccinated children

    For unvaccinated adolescents ages 11–12

    For adults at increased risk of infection (e.g. those attending STD clinics)

    Persons with a history of an STD

    Persons with multiple sexual partners

    Persons having sex with an injection-drug user

    Persons engaging in illegal drug use

    Household members, sex partners, drug-sharing partners of person with chronic HBV

Table 56-1 Interpretation of the hepatitis B panel

Test	Results	Interpretation
HBsAg	Negative	
anti-HBc	Negative	Susceptible
anti-HBs	Negative	
HBsAg	Negative	
anti-HBc	Positive	Immune due to natural infection
anti-HBs	Positive	
HBsAg	Negative	
anti-HBc	Negative	Immune due to hepatitis B vaccination
anti-HBs	Positive	
HBsAg	Positive	
anti-HBc	Positive	
anti-HBc IgM	Positive	Acutely infected
anti-HBs	Negative	
HBsAg	Positive	
anti-HBc	Positive	Chronically infected
anti-HBc Igm	Negative	
anti-HBs	Negative	
HBsAg	Negative	Four interpretations possible:
anti-HBc	Positive	(1) May be recovering from acute HBV infection
anti-HBs	Negative	(2) May distantly immune and test is not sensitive enough to detect very low level of anti-HBs in serum
		(3) May be susceptible with a false-positive anti-HBc
		(4) May be an undetectable level of HBsAg present in the serum and the person is actually a carrier

anti-HBc, hepatitis B core antibody; anti-HBc Igm, IgM antibody against HBc; anti-HBs, hepatitis B surface antibody; HBV, hepatitis B virus; HBsAg, hepatitis B surface antigen.
Used with permission from CDC viral hepatitis B. www.cdc.gov/ncidod/diseases/hepatitisb/Bserology.htm

Persons on hemodialysis, receiving blood clotting factor concentrates or occupational exposure to blood

Persons in drug treatment/long-term correctional facilities

Postexposure prophylaxis

Give hepatitis B immune globulin (HBIG) and vaccine to unvaccinated sex partners within 14 days of contact or when there has been exposure to person with acute hepatitis B

HEPATITIS C

The most common chronic bloodborne infection

Incubation period from 2 to 26 weeks (average 6–7 weeks)

Chronic infection develops in 80% after acute infection 65% have active liver disease

Patients are not clinically ill, so are not aware of illness and transmit to others

Transmission

Direct percutaneous exposure to infected blood

No association to medical, dental, surgical procedures or tattooing

Role of sexual activity is controversial

Diagnosis

Anti-HCV or HCV RNA

Management

Treatment

For chronic liver disease:

> Alpha interferon alone or in combination with oral agent ribavirin for 6–12 months

Prevention

No available vaccine

Persons seeking care for STDs

> Offer counseling/testing *if*

> (1) Illegal drug use even once or twice many years ago

> (2) Blood transfusion or solid organ transplant before July 1992

> (3) Receipt of clotting factor concentrates produced before 1987

> (4) Long-term hemodialysis

HERPES SIMPLEX VIRUS (HSV)

Genital herpes is a recurrent, life long viral infection

There are two types: HSV-1 and HSV-2, both can infect the genital tract

HSV-2 lesions more likely to recur than HSV-1

Presentation

Primary HSV:	Painful grouped vesicles may last up to a week
	Local pain, itching, dysuria
	Constitutional symptoms–fever, myalgia, malaise, headache
Recurrent HSV:	Vesicles or ulcers but no constitutional symptoms

Diagnosis

Appearance is typical but perform viral culture to confirm diagnosis

Serology is available, Only type-specific IgG-based assays should be requested

FDA approved IgG-based type-specific assays:

- POCkit HSV-2 (Diagnology)
- HerpeSelect-1 ELISA IgG or HerpeSelect-2 ELISA IgG (Focus Technology, Inc.)
- HerpeSelect 1 and 2 Immunoblot IgG (Focus Technology, Inc.)

Management

Pediatric/non-sexually active adolescent cases:

Sexual abuse must be considered as etiology

If history of oral cold sores and has Type 1 HSV, less likely to be secondary to sexual abuse; despite this, some type of investigation needs to be conducted by the healthcare provider or referral to appropriate child advocacy center to evaluate for and ensure there has been no inappropriate sexual contact (See Sexual abuse, Chapter 54)

Sexually active patient:

> Screen also for syphilis, gonorrhea and chlamydia, bacterial vaginosis and trichomonas – may be too tender at initial presentation to complete and may have to perform these tests at the follow-up visit after resolution of acute herpetic ulceration

Educate patient:

> Highest rate of transmission occurs with active lesions or during prodrome but virus can be transmitted in an asymptomatic state
>
> Herpetic and any ulcerative lesions may increase HIV transmission, offer HIV testing
>
> Refrain from oral sex when have a cold sore
>
> Use condoms at all times due to subclinical infections
>
> Abstain from any sexual activity during outbreaks
>
> Seek treatment at first sign of infection to decrease viral shedding
>
> HSV can be transmitted perinatally to infant, active outbreaks while pregnant patient in labor necessitate Cesarean delivery

Treatment

Pediatric cases

Acyclovir

> Only FDA approved medication for children under age of 18
>
> Infants: 20 mg/kg IV every 8 hours for 21 days for disseminated disease limited to skin and mucous membranes

Adolescent cases

First clinical episode:	Acyclovir 400 mg po tid for 7–10 days or
	Valacyclovir 1 g po bid for 7–10 days
Recurrent episodes:	Must initiate treatment within 1 day
	Acyclovir 400 mg po bid for 5 days *or*
	Acyclovir 800 mg po bid for 5 days *or*
	Valacyclovir 500 mg po bid for 5 days *or*
	Valacyclovir 1.0 g po once a day for 5 days

Suppressive therapy:	For 6 recurrences/year
	Periodically (once/year) discontinue treatment and reassess need for continuation
	Acyclovir 400 mg po bid *or*
	Famciclovir 250 mg po bid *or*
	Valacyclovir 500 mg po daily *or*
	Valacyclovir 1.0 g po daily

Immunocompromised individuals need specific dosing (www.cdc.gov)

Local care

Sitz baths tid to qid to keep area clean and enhance voiding

Avoid soaps

Increase po fluids to keep urine dilute and less irritating

May need to place indwelling catheter if urinary retention occurs

Use of topical 2% lidocaine gel to ulcerated areas may minimize burning with urination; discontinue if aggrevates symptoms

Narcotics, i.e. codeine may be needed for pain

HUMAN IMMUNODEFICIENCY VIRUS (HIV)

Key points

One-third to one-half of the new HIV infections each year are in people younger than age 25

Those with an STD are 2 to 5 times more likely to become infected with HIV if exposed

Syphilitic and herpetic ulcers increase the transmission of HIV by increasing blood–mucosal contact with sex

Gonorrhea and chlamydia facilitate transmission of HIV by increasing amount of viral shedding in genital secretions

Detection

Offer testing to:

(1) Young women seeking evaluation/testing for STDs

Medical/gynecologic conditions consistent with HIV-related illness

History of substance abuse associated with unprotected sex

History of survival sex or prostitution

Partner known to be HIV infected or at high risk

Victims of rape/sexual abuse (baseline and 3–9 months later)

History of STDs

History of pelvic inflammatory disease

Cervical dysplasia

Pregnancy

History of unprotected sex with multiple partners, older men or partner from area where HIV is prevalent

Patient desires testing

(2) Anyone with acute retroviral syndrome:

Fever, malaise, lymphadenopathy, skin rash within first few weeks of HIV infection before antibody test positive

- Perform HIV plasma RNA test
- A positive test should be confirmed with another HIV test; these patients may qualify for clinical trials and should be immediately referred to an HIV clinical care provider

Diagnosis

[Informed consent must be obtained before HIV test]

(1) If available in your clinical setting, OraQuick Rapid HIV-1 antibody test

Fingerstick test with results in 20 minutes

- A negative test requires no further testing
- Retest:

Persons with exposure within past 3 months

- A positive:

    Confirm with Western blot

    or

(2) Draw antibody to HIV-1/HIV-2 (enzyme immunoassay, EIA)

    (HIV Ab detectable 95% of patients within 3 months of exposure)

    IF reactive – Confirm with Western blot *or*

    - Immunofluorescence assay (IFA)

Management

(1) Refer patient immediately for initial counseling and behavioral, psychosocial and medical evaluation and treatment services

(2) Evaluate patient for symptoms or signs that suggest advance HIV infection (e.g. fever, weight loss, diarrhea, cough, shortness of breath, and oral candidiasis) – this should prompt urgent referral for medical care

(3) Encourage HIV positive patients to notify partners. Refer patient to health department partner-notification programs. If patient is unwilling to notify their partners, the health department should be informed to use confidential procedures to notify partners

(4) Draw hCG, ensure patient is not pregnant

Components of pretest HIV counseling for youth

See Table 56-2

Components of post-test HIV counseling

See Table 56-3

HUMAN PAPILLOMA VIRUS

See Condyloma acuminatum (Chapter 10)

NEISSERIA GONORRHOEAE

Can be associated with sexual abuse in children, typically those infected have a greenish vaginal discharge, it is rare to be asymptomatic

Table 56-2   Components of pretest HIV counseling for youth (provide over 1–3 visits)

Education about AIDS
Education about HIV infection (course, lack of cure, availability of treatment, asymptomatic infection, routes of transmission, window period)
Assessment of current and past sexual and substance-using behavior
Assessment of psychological history and supports
Screen for domestic violence
Risks and benefits of testing
Previous HIV testing dates and results, including home testing
Meaning of positive, negative and indeterminate test results
Availability of confidential and anonymous testing
Applicable protection of HIV-related information in record
Reporting requirements
Review of safe sex and other risk-reduction practices
Development of a personal plan for risk reduction and for protecting others
Discuss plans for disclosure and support during the testing process
Discuss and access impact of a positive test
Discuss implications of a positive test for pregnant women, strategies to reduce perinatal transmission
Describe care available
Assess and discuss need for testing of any living children, if the mother is positive
Obtain informed, non-coerced consent
Draw blood
Discuss need for retesting if recent possible exposure or unsafe behavior in the future
Schedule follow-up visit(s) for more pretest counseling and support if indicated
Schedule results visit (far enough in advance to allow confirmation of a positive test)

Used with permission from Samples CL. Human immunodeficiency virus in young women. In Emans SJ, Laufer MR, Goldstein DP, eds. *Pediatric and Adolescent Gynecology*, 4th edn. Philadelphia: Lippincott-Raven, 1998

Females aged 15–19 years at highest risk of acquiring infection

85% of infected women are asymptomatic, therefore screening of sexually active young women is critical

Gonorrhea can be transmitted via oral sex and cause pharyngitis

Patients infected with gonorrhea are often coinfected with chlamydia, leading to a recommendation that in some populations it is less expensive to treat chlamydia rather than test for it

Diagnosis

Pediatric cases

Culture is the gold-standard, DNA probe and PCR are not appropriate because of theoretic false positive results

Table 56-3   Components of post-test HIV counseling (always done in person, not by phone or letter)

Negative result
Explain result is ready
Give result, allow person to express feelings
Meaning of a negative result, review window period
Review personal protection plan and plans for notifying support person or
     partner
Reassess risk, including risky behavior since the test was done (if any)
Plan and schedule for retesting after window interval, if indicated
Discuss documentation of test result and release of test information
Stress a negative test does not confer immunity or protection

Positive result
Review psychosocial needs with care team prior to visit, have crisis intervention plan
     in place
When patient arrives, explain result is ready
Give result, allow person to express feelings, give comfort and listen
Reassess emotional state and need for support, offer to involve family or support
     person, if patient chooses
Reassure that treatment, care, support are available, that HIV infection is a chronic
     disease
Discuss importance of follow-up and education, and schedule follow-up
     appointment as soon as possible, assuming patient will retain little of what you
     discuss today
Stress hope, optimism, availability of support (hotline, support groups)
Review how to avoid transmission, reinfection
Review self-care plan to monitor immune function and stay healthy (lifestyle,
     nutrition, substance use)
If pregnant, rediscuss options, including treatment options to reduce transmission,
     impact of HIV on prenatal care
Reassess reproductive health care plans (contraception, plans for children, etc.)
Begin or schedule baseline assessment

Indeterminate result
Give result, allow person to react
Review meaning of an indeterminate result (may be caused by other conditions,
     seroconversion)
Stress need to continue risk-reduction plan
Schedule follow-up test in 3–6 months
Evaluate clinically for evidence of recent infection, other conditions
If pregnant, repeat test immediately, consider viral culture or polymerase chain reaction
test, consult with HIV infectious disease expert

Used with permission from Samples CL. Human immunodeficiency virus in young women.
In Emans SJ, Laufer MR, Goldstein DP, eds. *Pediatric and Adolescent Gynecology*, 4th edn. Philadelphia:
Lippincott-Raven, 1998

Adolescent cases

Culture

DNA probe

PCR (urine or endocervical)

Management

Pediatric cases

Gonorrhea in a pediatric patient is secondary to sexual abuse patient must be treated and referred for a sexual abuse evaluation (see Sexual abuse, Chapter 54)

Adolescent cases

Educate patient that short of abstinence, condom use for anal, vaginal and oral sex is the most effective way to prevent disease

Stress need for routine screening, including screening for gonorrhea with each new sexual partner which should be repeated 4–6 weeks after treatment for gonorrhea to test for reinfection

Treatment

Pediatric cases:

> Ceftriaxone 125 mg IM in a single dose *or*
>
> Spectinomycin 40 mg/kg (max 2 g) IM single dose

Children > 45 kg and > than 8 years of age can be treated as adults:

> Ceftriaxone 125 mg IM in a single dose *or*
>
> *Ciprofloxacin 500 mg orally in a single dose *or*
>
> IF chlamydia not ruled out add
>
> - Azithromycin 1 g orally in a single dose *or*
> - Doxycycline 100 mg orally twice a day for 7 days

*Teens > 45 kg can be treated with quinolones

*Quinolones should not be used for infections from Asia/the Pacific including Hawaii

Follow-up

Instruct patient to have partner referred for evaluation/treatment

Avoid intercourse until therapy complete and have no further symptoms and until partner is treated and is without symptoms

SYPHILIS

Key points

Systemic disease caused by *Treponema pallidum*

Syphilis facilitates transmission of HIV therefore screening and treatment have a public health benefit

Many teens may have had undetected chancres and not be a aware of infectivity, therefore screening for at-risk teen is important

Screen annually:	Persons who exchange sex for money
	Persons with multiple partners
	Persons with partners who exchange sex for money
	Persons admitted to jails
	Illicit users of drugs
	Persons with two other STDs

Natural history of disease

Stage 1: Primary syphilis	Non-tender ulcer or chancre at site of inoculation within 3 weeks of exposure
	Often undetected because non-tender
Stage 2: Secondary syphilis	Occurs within weeks to months
	Malaise, fever, headache, adenopathy
	Maculopapular rash involves palms/soles
Stage 3: Tertiary syphilis	Final stage takes years to develop
	Neurologic, cardiovascular, skeletal abnormalities
Latent syphilis:	Syphilis detected with serology but lacking clinical manifestations

Early latent: Acquired within preceding year with:

documented seroconversion

unequivocal symptoms of primary or secondary disease

partner with primary, secondary or early latent syphilis

Late latent: Syphilis not meeting above criteria or for unknown duration

NOTE: Patients with latent syphilis need clinical assessment for tertiary disease (e.g. aortitis, gummas, iritis) and need CSF exam if:

- neuro/eye signs/symptom
- evidence tertiary disease
- treatment failure
- HIV infection

Diagnosis

Perform:

Darkfield examination of lesion exudates

Direct fluorescent antibody test of lesion exudates

And/or serologic testing with:

- Venereal Disease Research Laboratory (VDRL) *or*
- Rapid Plasma Reagin (RPR)

    IF positive: Confirm with treponemal test Fluorescent treponemal antibody absorbed (FTA-ABS)

- Non-treponemal tests (VDRL or RPR)

    *Titers correlate with disease activity

    A four-fold change in titer (change in 2 dilutions) is required to demonstrate clinical difference between tests

    (e.g. from 1:16 to 1:4 or 1:8 to 1:32)

    *VDRL and RPR titers are not equal

    Therefore, use the same test to follow patient response to treatment

Management

NOTE All patients with syphilis should be tested for HIV infection and screened for other STDs including: gonorrhea, chlamydia, trichomonas

Pediatric cases

Infants with syphilis require maternal evaluation to assess for congenital vs acquired infection; treatment is based on neonatal titer vs the maternal titer. For complete evaluation and treatment consult with CDC (www.cdc.gov) Children who are identified as having reactive serologic tests for syphilis > 1 month of age, need maternal serology and records reviewed to distinguish congenital vs acquired syphilis. For complete evaluation and treatment guidelines consult with CDC (www.cdc.gov)

Pediatric syphilis cases other than case of vertical transmission require a sexual abuse evaluation

Adolescent cases

Educate about spread of disease by contact with ulcers, chancres, condylomata and need for condom use

Treatment

Adolescent cases:

Primary/secondary syphilis:	Benzathine penicillin G 2.4 million units IM in a single dose
	IF penicillin allergy:
	Doxycycline 100 mg orally twice daily for 14 days *or*
	Tetracycline 500 mg orally four times daily for 14 days
Latent syphilis:	
Early latent:	Benzathine penicillin G 2.4 million units IM in a single dose
Late latent:	Benzathine penicillin G 7.2 million units total, given as three doses of 2.4 million units each at 1-week intervals
	IF penicillin allergy:
	Doxycycline 100 mg orally twice daily for 28 days *or*
	Tetracycline 500 mg orally four times daily for 28 days

Tertiary syphilis: Benzathine penicillin G 7.2 million units total, given as three doses of 2.4 million units IM each at 1-week intervals

Follow-up

Primary/secondary syphilis: Re-examine clinically and with serology at 6 and 12 months

Sustained fourfold increase in VDRL/RPR is a failed treatment or reinfection

- Test for HIV

- Retreat, see www.cdc.gov

Latent syphilis: Repeat VDRL/RPR at 6, 12 and 24 months

Retreat IF

- Titers increase fourfold

- High initial titer (1:32) fails to decline fourfold within 12-24 months

- Signs/symptoms develop

Management of sexual contacts

Primary, secondary, early latent:

Treat those exposed within 90 days presumptively

- Those exposed > 90 days, treat on serology or presumptively if follow-up is uncertain

Late latent

- Evaluate partners clinically/serologically

TRICHOMONAS

See Vulvovaginitis, Chapter 69

BIBLIOGRAPHY

www.cdc.gov

Centers for Disease Control and Prevention. Sexually transmitted diseases treatment guidelines 2002. *MMWR* 2002;51(No. RR-6).

Killebrew M, Garofalo R. Talking to teens about sex, sexuality, and sexually transmitted infections. *Pediatr Ann* 2002;31:566–72

Samples CL. Human immunodeficiency virus in young women. In Emans SJ, Laufer MR, Goldstein DP, eds. *Pediatric and Adolescent Gynecology,* 4th edn. Philadelphia: Lippincott-Raven, 1998:531–52

57 Substance abuse

Tobacco, alcohol and marijuana are still the most widely used substances by children and adolescents

Drug use in adolescence is one of the strongest predictors of lifetime development of drug dependence

Education at an early age (by age 10) about the negative effects of specific substances is essential to prevention

RISK FACTORS

Family factors

    Family history of substance use, dependence or both

    Dysfunctional parenting style

    Extreme permissiveness or authoritarianism

    Conflicted families

Problem behaviors

    Antisocial behavior

    Negative affect, low adaptability, and impulsivity

    Aggressiveness

    Early sexual experience

    Attention deficit disorder (ADD)

School factors

    Early school failure

    Incomplete homework and truancy

    Lack of commitment to education

Association with substance using peers

Early onset of substance use

History of sexual abuse

Community factors

Ready availability of alcohol and other drugs

Tolerance for the use of alcohol or illegal drugs

Overpopulated, disorganized, and deteriorating neighborhoods

TOBACCO

Identification

Nicotine usually the first substance abused

Initiation associated with:

Low socioeconomic status

Low level of parent education

Ages 11–16

Protective factors:

Close communication with parents

Positive parental support, high self-esteem

Assertiveness, social competence, school success, regular church attendance, and strong sense of right and wrong

Intervention

A 'no-smoking office' with appropriate signs, magazines without tobacco advertising, and tobacco-free posters, literature and referral

Sources

National Institute of Health/US Public Service guidelines to address tobacco use in children and adolescents:

(1) Anticipate: Provide age-appropriate education to parents and children. Compliment youth who are nonsmokers

(2) Ask: Inquire about environmental exposure (ETS) and tobacco use by parents, children, and youth and record it prominently in the patient's chart or in the problem list

(3) Advise: Use clear, personal, relevant messages to advise parents and youth who use tobacco to quit

(4) Assess: If the tobacco user is ready to quit. Use motivational interviewing techniques and repetition to encourage those not yet ready to quit to consider quitting. Emphasize causal relation with reproductive cancers; thromboembolic events with estrogen containing contraceptives; pregnancy-associated risks, i.e. ectopic pregnancy, low birth weight infants

(5) Arrange follow-up: Schedule follow-up visits to enhance the motivation to quit and to provide encouragement and help with relapse prevention for those who have successfully quit.

Those who smoke 10 or more cigarettes a day may benefit from nicotine replacement therapy and perhaps bupropion hydrochloride in conjunction with behavioral techniques but data is limited in adolescents

Parents should be encouraged to be role models

Concurrent screening and treatment for other substance use

ALCOHOL AND MARIJUANA

Identification

Alcoholism should be suspect in young people who are often intoxicated or experience withdrawal symptoms from chronic or recurrent alcohol use; those who tolerate large quantities of alcohol; those who attempt unsuccessfully to cut down or stop alcohol use; those who experience blackouts attributable to drinking; or those who continue drinking despite adverse social, educational, occupational, physical, or psychological consequences or alcohol-related injuries

Alcoholism should be suspect in young people who have a family history of alcoholism

Marijuana should be suspect in those with decreasing cognitive function particularly short-term memory

CRAFFT test: screens for alcohol and other drug abuse with questions developmentally appropriate for teenagers. A score of 2 or higher indicates risk. A score of 4 or higher should raise suspicion of substance dependence:

C Have you ever found yourself in a CAR driven by someone (including yourself) who was 'high' or had been using alcohol or drugs?

R Do you ever use alcohol or drugs to RELAX, feel better about yourself, fit in?

A Do you ever use alcohol or drugs while you are by yourself, ALONE?

F Do you ever FORGET things you did while using alcohol or drugs?

F Do your FAMILY or FRIENDS ever tell you that you should cut down on your drinking or drug use?

T Have you ever gotten into TROUBLE while you were using alcohol or drugs?

Intervention

Treatment resources for adolescents are scarce yet limited data indicate they are effective. Check with local health or law enforcement agencies for the services in your area

Treatment of adolescents requires a broadened scope of services, including family interventions, mental health care, remedial education, vocational habilitation, and community outreach

OTHER SUBSTANCES INCREASING IN ABUSE BY ADOLESCENTS

Club drugs on the rise:

- Ecstasy (MDMA)
- Gamma-hydroxybutyrate (GHB, liquid X, g-juice)
- Rohypnol (roofies, forget pill)
- Ketamine (Special K, Vitamin K, Kit Kat)
- Can lead to hallucinations, permanent memory loss, thought difficulty and mood changes

Inhalants (volatile hydrocarbons like toluene, gasoline, solvents, glue, spray paint) cause seizures, hypoxemia and arrythmias

Heroin with increased purity available leads to more deaths

LSD and PCP can lead to violence

Metamphetamine (crystal meth, ice or crank) causes violence, hallucinations and memory loss

INTERNET RESOURCES

www.health.org

www.theantidrug.com

BIBLIOGRAPHY

American Academy of Pediatrics. Indications for management and referral of patients involved in substance abuse. *Pediatrics* 2000;106:143–8

American College of Obstetricians and Gynecologists. *Tool Kit For Teen Care* 2003

Knight JR, Sherritt L, Shrier LA, *et al*. Validity of the CRAFFT substance abuse screening test among adolescent clinic patients. *Arch Pediatr Adolesc Med* 2002;156:607–14

Mee-Lee D. *Adolescent Crosswalk. American Society of Addiction Medicine Patient Placement Criteria for the Treatment of Substance-Related Disorders*. 2nd edn. Chevy Chase, MD: ASAM, 1998

Schonberg SK, ed. *Substance Abuse: A Guide for Health Professionals*. Elk Grove Village, IL: American Academy of Pediatrics, 1988

Stein RJ, Haddock CK, OByrne K *et al*. The pediatrician's role in reducing tobacco exposure in children. *Pediatrics* 2000;106:E66

58 Toxic shock syndrome (TSS)

An illness characterized by high fever, sunburn-like rash, desquamation, hypotension, and abnormalities in multiple organ systems

Syndrome associated with a focal infection (e.g. infected wound, abscess, vaginal colonization with *Staphylococcus aureus*)

S. aureus bacteria produce a toxic shock syndrome toxin (TSST-1) that leads to clinical development of TSS

Syndrome has been associated with continuous tampon use

Peak occurrence in menstruating women on 4th day of menses

TSS has increased with female barrier contraceptive use (e.g. diaphragm use) but is still relatively rare. If prior history of TSS, patient not candidate for diaphragm use for contraception

Menstrual-associated TSS has decreased since the FDA instituted standardized absorbency labeling of tampons and encouraged users to use the lowest absorbency tampon compatible for their flow

(Probable when 4 of 5 of the following present)

Fever of 38.9°C or higher

Rash: diffuse macular erythroderma (looks like sunburn)

Desquamation 1 to 2 weeks after the onset of the illness, particularly of the palms and soles

Hypotension (systolic blood pressure ≤ 90 mmHg for 16 years and older, or below fifth percentile by age for children under 16 years, or orthostatic decrease ≥ 15 mmHg in diastolic blood pressure or orthostatic syncope or orthostatic dizziness

Involvement of three or more of the following organ systems:

- Gastrointestinal (vomiting or diarrhea)
- Muscular (severe myalgia or creatinine phosphokinase (CPK) level at least two times upper limit of normal)
- Mucous membranes (vaginal, oropharyngeal, or conjunctival) hyperemia
- Renal (blood urea nitrogen or creatinine at least two times the upper limit of normal or > 5 leukocytes/high power field in the absence of urinary tract infection
- Hepatic (total bilirubin, AST, ALT at least two times the upper limit of normal)
- Hematologic (platelet count < 100 000/mm^3)
- Central nervous system (disorientation or alterations in consciousness when fever and hypotension are absent)

MANAGEMENT

Acute

Adolescents with the above symptoms must remove tampon and go to the emergency room as disease progresses rapidly

Hospitalize patient and treat for shock with IV fluid resuscitation

Order complete blood count, complete metabolic profile, coagulation tests, CPK level

- Hypocalcemia, hypomagnesemia, elevated CPK are common

Perform vaginal exam and remove tampon if not already removed

- Gram stain vaginal pool

Culture blood, rectum, vagina, oropharynx, anterior nares and urine

Order serology for Rocky Mountain spotted fever, leptospirosis, measles

- (Must return negative to diagnose TSS)

Administer penicillinase-resistant antistaphylococcal antibiotics for 2 weeks, initially intravenously and with improvement can transition to oral to complete 2 weeks of therapy

Follow-up

Recurrence rate of 30%

Presence of antibody to TSST-1 is reassuring

Avoid tampons for 6 months

After 6 months

- Avoid superabsorbent tampons
- Tampons should be matched to amount of menstrual flow

    A tampon is too absorbent if:

    The tampon is hard to remove

    Vaginal dryness occurs

    The tampon shreds on removal

    The tampon doesn't need to be removed after several hours

- Use tampons intermittently with pad use at night
- Change tampons every 4–6 hours
- Remove tampons and call a physician should vomiting, diarrhea, rash or fever occur

BIBLIOGRAPHY

Emans SJ. Vulvovaginal complaints in the adolescent. In Emans SJ, Laufer MR, Goldstein DP, eds. *Pediatric and Adolescent Gynecology*, 4th edn. Philadelphia: Lippincott-Raven, 1998:447–9

Kwitkowski VE. Demko SG. Infectious disease emergencies in primary care. *Lippincott's Prim Care Practice* 1999;3:108–25

Nakase JY. Update on emerging infections from the Centers for Disease Control and Prevention. *Ann Emerg Med* 2000;36:268–69

Schwartz B, Gaventa S, Bromme CV, *et al*. Nonmenstrual toxic shock syndrome associated with barrier contraceptives: report of a case-controlled study. *Rev Infect Dis* 1989;11:S43

Tofte RW, Williams DN. Toxic shock syndrome. Evidence of a broad clinical spectrum. *J Am Med Assoc* 1981;246:2163–7

59 Tubal mass

TYPES

Prepubertal:

> Very rare
>
> If simple, cyst
>
> If complex, torsion (see Ovarian/adnexal torsion, Chapter 39)

Postmenarcheal:

> Ectopic pregnancy
>
> If simple, cyst
>
> If complex: torsion (see Ovarian/adnexal torsion, Chapter 39), hydrosalpinx, endosalpingiosis

DIAGNOSIS AND TREATMENT

Prepubertal:

> Ultrasound
>
> Laparoscopy (see Operative care, Chapter 37)

Postmenarchal:

> Pregnancy test, sexually transmitted disease (STD) testing and pelvic exam in the sexually active adolescent
>
> Laparoscopy if above tests negative and signs/symptoms warrant surgical evaluation (see Operative care, Chapter 37 for technique)
>
> - IF endosalpingiosis, consider GnRH agonist suppressive therapy for six months followed by continuous hormonal suppression; suggested association with chronic pelvic pain and endometriosis (see Endometriosis, Chapter 18 for dosing)
>
> IF positive for PID by STD and/or pelvic, treat as inpatient (see Pelvic inflammatory disease, Chapter 43) as theorectically better penetration of fallopian tubes with IV antibiotics

- IF antibiotics successful and becomes asymptomatic, would monitor for increased growth. If stable, would postpone removal unless difficulty with conception. Warning instructions for ectopic pregnancy

IF positive for pregnancy, presume ectopic pregnancy

- Treat conservatively with surgery: laparoscopy, prefer salpingostomy to salpingectomy *or*
- Medical: methotrexate

Methotrexate management for ectopic pregnancy

Exclusion criteria

Significant hemoperitoneum (> 3 cm diameter pocket of fluid)

Evidence of impending rupture

Sonographic evidence of extrauterine fetal activity

Adnexal mass greater or equal to 3.5 cm

Beta-human chorionic gonadotropin (βhCG) greater than 6000 IU/ml (IRP-International Reference Panel)

Declining βhCG levels (40% drop from prior level within 3 days)

Evidence of hepatic, renal or hematologic abnormalities: Liver function tests greater or equal to 1.5 × normal; creatinine > 1.5 mg/dl; platelets < 100 000 mm^3; white blood cell count < 3500 cells/μl; hematocrit < 34%

Co-existing intrauterine pregnancy

Inability to consent patient

Inability to comply with proper follow-up

Pretreatment laboratory tests

Complete blood count (CBC)

Blood type/Rh factor

ALT/AST

Quantitative hCG

Creatinine

Vaginal ultrasound or previous laparoscopy

Pathology from Karmen Biopsy or D&C if hCG less than or equal to 3000 IU/ml (IRP) and vaginal ultrasound negative

Medication dosing

(See Figure 59-1)

Height and weight in cm and kg then calculate body surface area (BSA) as m^2

Methotrexate dose of 50 mg/m^2 is calculated to nearest 10 mg increment given IM

Rho (D) immune globulin (RhoGAM) is given if Rh negative (300 g IM)

Follow-ups

(See Figure 59-2 for Patient consent, see Figure 59-3 for Patient instructions, and see Figure 59-4 Worksheet)

Day 0: Day of injection

Day 4: Quantitative(Q) hCG and abdominal exam; hCG may increase but exam should be same as pretreatment

Day 7: QhCG and CBC and abdominal exam:

CBC and abdominal exam should be the same as pretreatment

QhCG should decline greater than or equal to 15% of Day 4 QhCG, then follow QhCG weekly, expecting 15% drop from previous levels until negative; discuss contraception

IF QHCG does not decline 15%, then perform laparoscopy or retreat with methotrexate

- Retreatment is followed by recheck QhCG on days 11 and 14 with expected decrease of greater than or equal to 15% of day 11; if still fails go to laparoscopy

- Laparoscopy: if no findings do D&C; if findings, treatment conservative, salpingostomy if possible

IF patient presents with pelvic/abdominal pain during course of treatment, assess clinically and check by ultrasound and CBC. If acute abdomen, surgical therapy

Ensure that chemotherapy spill kit is available at the site where methotrexate is given. Obtain from pharmacy

University OB/GYN Associates, P.S.C.
601 South Floyd St., Suite 300
Louisville, KY 40202

METHOTREXATE DOSING CHART

Use 3cc syringe and any dosage above 2cc must be divided in two syringes and given as two IM injections.

SURFACE AREA (m²)	MILLIGRAM (mg)	MILLILITER (cc)
2.60	130.0mg	5.2cc
2.55	127.5mg	5.1cc
2.50	125.0mg	5.0cc
2.45	122.5mg	4.9cc
2.40	120.0mg	4.8cc
2.35	117.5mg	4.7cc
2.30	115.0mg	4.6cc
2.25	112.5mg	4.5cc
2.20	110.0mg	4.4cc
2.15	107.5mg	4.3cc
2.10	105.0mg	4.2cc
2.05	102.5mg	4.1cc
2.00	100.0mg	4.0cc
1.95	97.5mg	3.9cc
1.90	95.0mg	3.8cc
1.85	92.5mg	3.7cc
1.80	90.0mg	3.6cc
1.75	87.5mg	3.5cc
1.70	85.0mg	3.4cc
1.65	82.5mg	3.3cc
1.60	80.0mg	3.2cc
1.55	77.5mg	3.1cc
1.50	75.0mg	3.0cc
1.45	72.5mg	2.9cc
1.40	70.0mg	2.8cc
1.35	67.5mg	2.7cc
1.30	65.0mg	2.6cc
1.25	62.5mg	2.5cc
1.20	60.0mg	2.4cc
1.15	57.5mg	2.3cc
1.10	55.0mg	2.2cc
1.05	52.5mg	2.1cc
1.00	50.0mg	2.0cc
.95	47.5mg	1.9cc
.90	45.0mg	1.8cc
.85	42.5mg	1.7cc

Figure 59-1   Medication dosing chart for methotrexate treatment

INFORMED CONSENT FOR USE OF INTRAMUSCULAR METHOTREXATE IN THE TREATMENT OF UNRUPTURED ECTOPIC PREGNANCY

You have been diagnosed as having a high probability of having an unruptured ectopic (tubal) pregnancy. A pregnancy located in the tube if left untreated can rupture, resulting in internal bleeding, shock, and rarely death.

Traditionally, treatment for tubal pregnancy has been either surgical removal of the fallopian tube or surgical removal of the tubal pregnancy from the tube with preservation of the fallopian tube. However, several centers in the United States and abroad have recently begun treating selected patients with tubal pregnancy with an anti-cancer drug called Methotrexate to dissolve the tubal pregnancy, and thus avoid surgery. This drug has been employed in the treatment of pregnancy-related tumors for over 40 years with excellent results and without lasting effects to either the patient or later pregnancies.

Your doctor has determined that you would benefit from Methotrexate treatment of your tubal pregnancy. If you consent to Methotrexate treatment, the drug will be administered in the office as an intramuscular injection at a dose calculated for your individual height and weight. Prior to treatment, it will be necessary to obtain some blood tests and an ultrasound to check the size of the pregnancy and to make sure that your blood count, kidney and liver functions are normal.

A small number of patients require additional doses of Methotrexate to completely remove the ectopic pregnancy. This will be determined by the rate at which pregnancy hormone levels fall. Occasionally, medical treatment with Methotrexate is unsuccessful.

IT IS IMPORTANT TO REMEMBER THAT EVEN THOUGH YOU HAVE RECEIVED METHOTREXATE, A TUBAL RUPTURE CAN STILL OCCUR AND THAT EMERGENCY SURGERY MAY BE REQUIRED. Therefore, you should contact your doctor *immediately* if you develop abdominal pain.

After receiving the medication, it will be necessary to have blood drawn for pregnancy hormone testing. Blood will be drawn twice during the first week after Methotrexate therapy. If the levels are dropping appropriately, blood pregnancy hormone levels will subsequently be tested once per week until the blood tests are negative. A negative blood test means that there is no further evidence of any active pregnancy tissue. At this point, no further tests will be required.

Even if your tubal pregnancy totally resolves on Methotrexate treatment, scarring may occur in your tube as a result of tubal pregnancy, and this could cause you to have later tubal pregnancies and/or subsequent infertility.

The side effects of this drug are minimal. They include ulcer-like sores in the mouth and a stinging sensation in the eyes. These side effects usually become apparent about one week after you receive the medication and may last for about one week. You may also feel quite tired during the week after therapy, but if you feel up to it you may resume normal activity, including going back to work.

Do not drink alcohol for two weeks after receiving Methotrexate, since alcohol can cause liver damage to those who receive Methotrexate. Do not take aspirin-like compounds like Advil or Motrin for two to three weeks after receiving Methotrexate.

You should avoid excess exposure to sun or use of sunlamps for four weeks following Methotrexate therapy because your skin may be more sensitive to sunlight than usual and burn excessively.

(Continued)

Figure 59-2   Patient consent form for methotrexate treatment

Figure 59-2 (*Continued*)

The nature and purpose of Methotrexate therapy for my ectopic pregnancy has been fully explained. I fully understand the potential benefits and possible risks of the proposed treatment, the likelihood of serious problems without treatment, and the available alternatives.

I am aware that other unexpected risks or complications not discussed may occur and that no guarantees or promises have been made to made concerning the results of any procedure or treatment. I also understand that during the course of the proposed treatment, unforeseen conditions may be revealed, requiring the performance of additional procedures, and I authorize such procedures to be performed.

My signature below constitutes my acknowledgment that 1) I understand this consent form, 2) such procedures have been satisfactorily explained to me and I have all the information that I desire and 3) I hereby authorize my physician to give me Methotrexate in an attempt to dissolve my ectopic pregnancy.

_____   _____
Patient's name (please print)   Physician's signature

_____   _____
Patient's signature   Date

_____   _____
Parent's signature (if less than age 18)   Date

_____   _____
Witness

PATIENT INSTRUCTIONS FOLLOWING
I.M. METHOTREXATE ADMINISTRATION

- **Do not drink alcohol for two weeks after receiving Methotrexate**, since alcohol can cause liver damage in patients who received Methotrexate.
- **Do not take aspirin or aspirin-like compounds like Advil or Motrin for two to three weeks after receiving Methotrexate.** Take only Tylenol (that is, acetaminophen containing medications) as needed.
- **You should avoid excess exposure to sun or use of sunlamps for four weeks following Methotrexate therapy,** because your skin may be more sensitive to sunlight than usual and burn excessively.
- **Avoid pelvic exams and intercourse until complete resolution of ectopic pregnancy (undetectable pregnancy blood level).**
- **You should use birth control for the next 2 months.**
- **Avoid vitamin preparations containing Folic Acid.**

- -
- -

A blood pregnancy level (B-hCG) needs to be checked in 4 days and in 7 days by your doctor.

Please return on _____ (day 4) and on _____ (day 7) to have a B-hCG drawn. You should have these follow up tests drawn at one of our ambulatory blood drawing centers or at your doctor's office – **NOT IN THE EMERGENCY DEPARTMENT.**

If day 4 or 7 falls on a weekend, you can have your blood drawn at the Emergency Department by calling the gynecology resident at 562-3094. Day 4 titer may be either higher or lower than the current B-hCG level.

You will likely experience some crampy abdominal pain (4–7). Please notify your doctor if this occurs.

Call your doctor immediately or return to the Emergency Department for any moderate or severe pain, bleeding or weakness.

Figure 59-3   Patient instructions following IM methotrexate administration

METHOTREXATE PATIENT FORM

DATE —————————————— Doctor ——————————————

Patient Name —————————————— Age ————— Birth Date————

Address ———————————— City ————— State ———— Zip————

Phone #1 ( ) ————— Phone #2 ( ) ——————— Social Security No. ————

Hospital Number: ————————— Height ————— Weight —————

Date of Methotrexate 50mg/m^2: RX#1 ——————— -Dose ————

Date of Methotrexate 50mg/m^2: RX#1 ——————— -Dose ————— (if needed)

Laboratory Tests	Day 0 Initial Rx Date	Day 4 1st Post Rx Date	Day 7 2nd Post Rx Date	Day 11 (opt'1) 3rd Post Rx Date	Day 14 4th Post Rx Date
CBC					
Rh/Blood Type					
Quant hCG					
Serum creatinine					
ALT/AST					

US: Is a mass present?   Y - N

   Size   2 cm or more
          6 cm or less

Pathology:

Figure 59-4   Worksheet for methotrexate treatment

BIBLIOGRAPHY

Lipscomb GH, Stovall TG, Ling FW. Nonsurgical treatment of ectopic pregnancy. *N Eng J Med* 2000;342:1325–9

Stovall TG, Ling FW. Single dose methotrexate treatment. *Am J Obstet Gynecol* 1993;168:1759–65

60 Turner syndrome (TS)

DEFINITION

A chromosomal disorder caused by complete or partial X monosomy in some or all cells, often characterized by short stature and gonadal dysgenesis

KEY POINTS

Consider diagnosis of TS in:

Any female patient with:

- Unexplained growth failure or pubertal delay

Newborns with:

- Edema of hands/feet
- Nuchal folds
- Left-sided cardiac anomalies

    Coarctation of the aorta

    Hypoplastic left heart

- Low hairline/low set ears/small mandible

Children with:

- Short stature with declining growth velocity

    (< 10 centile for age)

- Elevated follicle stimulating hormone (FSH) level
- Any of the following:

    Cubitus valgus

    Nail hypoplasia

    Hyperconvex uplifted nails

    Multiple pigmented nevi

Characteristic facies

Short 4th metacarpal

High arched palate

Adolescents with:

- Absence of breast development by age 13
- Pubertal arrest
- Primary or secondary amenorrhea with elevated FSH
- Unexplained short stature

DIAGNOSIS

If suspect Turner syndrome – draw peripheral blood karyotype

If peripheral karyotype normal and still suspect TS, assess karyotype of additional tissue site (e.g. skin)

MANAGEMENT

Obtain cardiac evaluation/complete physical and echocardiogram:

- Congenital heart defect in 30% of TS patients

  Bicuspid aortic valve 30–50% cases

  Coarctation of aorta – 30% cases

  Aortic root dilation – < 5%

- IF cardiovascular malformation present

  Patient should be followed by cardiologist

  Subacute bacterial endocarditis prophylaxis indicated

- IF initial cardiac workup negative

  Repeat cardiac evaluation/echo at age 12–15 years

  Reevaluate aortic root

Obtain evaluation renal anomaly with renal ultrasound:

- Congenital renal malformations in 30% cases TS

  Rotational abnormalities

  Double collecting systems

  May have increased risk of hypertension, urinary tract infection hydronephrosis

- IF abnormality detected

    Refer for urologic care

    Repeat ultrasound/urine cultures every 3–5 years

Treat short stature:

- Consultation recommended with pediatric endocrinology
- Initiation of growth hormone (GH) indicated if growth below 5th centile
- Therapy can be started as early as age 2 years
- Use growth hormone (GH) until satisfactory height is attained or until bone age is > 14 years and patient's height has increased by < 2 cm over past year

Manage pubertal onset:

- 90% of TS patients have gonadal failure
- Individualize use of estrogen therapy to initiate/complete pubertal development/coordinate with pediatric endocrinology
- If growth promotion a priority, do not initiate estrogen before age 12 years unless height is maximized
- Estrogen therapy should be started by age 15 years
- Initiate estrogen at ¼ to 1/6th of the adult dose and increase every 3–6 months adding a progestin with 1st vaginal bleed or after 12–24 months of estrogen

    medroxyprogesterone acetate 10 mg days 16–25 or on low dose combination oral contraceptive (if not contraindicated by associated medical conditions)

- Low dose oral contraceptive pills may be contraindicated depending on associated anomalies (i.e. cardiac)

Yearly evaluation

Evaluate blood pressure:

- Hypertension common even in absence of cardiac/renal anomalies

Evaluate thyroid function:

- 10–30% develop primary hypothyroidism
- Measure thyroid stimulating hormone and total or free thyroxine every 1–2 years

Watch for hearing and speech deficits/and recurrent otitis:

- 30–40% TS patients have outer ear malformation/low set ears
- Early and aggressive treatment of otitis
- Refer to ENT/speech therapist for speech problems

Vision:

- Ophthamologic evaluation
- Strabismus/amblyopia and ptosis common

Orthopedic exam:

- Increased risk of congenital hip dislocation/scoliosis

Weight:

- Tendency for obesity

Watch for lymphedema:

- Can be controlled with support stockings/diuretics

For more information: www.turner-syndrome-us.org

BIBLIOGRAPHY

Saenger P, Albertson W, Conway GS, *et al*. Recommendations for the diagnosis and management of Turner syndrome. *J Clin Endocrinol Metab* 2001;86:3061

61 Urethral prolapse

ETIOLOGY

Unclear; probably related to a hypoestrogenic state

DIAGNOSIS

Symptoms: prepubertal vaginal bleeding, dysuria, frequency, urinary retention

Physical examination

(See Figure 61-1)

Initially: 2–3 cm large ulcerative doughnut shaped mass obscuring the urethra that is often bleeding or friable

After medical treatment: redundant pink estrogenized urethral meatus without bleeding or friability

MANAGEMENT

Estrogen cream: small amount to the area bid after a sitz bath with good air drying, no rubbing (candidal overgrowth can result with estrogen placed in a moist area)

Bleeding usually resolves within one week, with majority of the prolapse reduced within two weeks

Occasionally there will remain a prominent but uninflamed tissue

Rarely does the tissue become symptomatic again and if so repeat course of estrogen

If the child continues to have urinary retention after medical treatment, surgical intervention may need to be considered

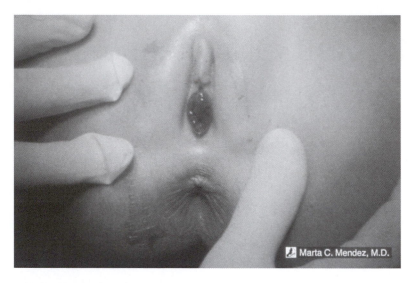

Figure 61-1 Urethral prolapse in a prepubertal girl. Used with permission from the North American Society for Pediatric and Adolescent Gynecology. *The Pedigyn Teaching Slide Set*. Elaine E. Yordan, MD (ed)

Excision

(Consult with pediatric urology/surgery)

Place foley cathether in the bladder

Excise the prolapse at the base

Interrupted 4-0 Vicryl sutures to approximate the urethral mucosa to the periurethral vestibular mucosa

Very vascular lesion; hemostasis is essential

Remove foley catheter in operating room

Send home on sitz baths and topical estrogen cream for another week

62 Urinary tract infection (UTI)

KEY POINTS

Recurrent urinary tract infection may be an indicator of renal disease

DIAGNOSIS

History

Onset of symptoms

Sexual activity

- Age at first intercourse
- Most recent sexual intercourse
- Urethral symptoms in male partner

Previous UTIs (culture documented or not)

Internal dysuria (abdominal pain with urination) – think UTI

External dysuria (pain when urine touches the external genitalia) – think vulvar cause (e.g. herpes)

Laboratory evaluation

Urinalysis

Urine culture/sensitivity

Wet preparation of vaginal discharge

IF sexually active, screen endocervix or urine for gonorrhea and chlamydia

MANAGEMENT

Instruct about improved voiding habits:

Void at least 3 to 5 times per day

Urinate with legs apart to prevent reflux of urine into vagina

Avoid use of bubble baths or irritants to the perineum

If sexually active, void after intercourse

Treatment

Infants < 2 months of age:

- Amoxicillin 20–40 mg/kg/day divided q 8 h orally for 7 days

Pediatric cases:

- Bactrim® (based on the trimethoprim component) 8–10 mg/kg/day divided q 12 h orally for 7 days

Adolescents:

- If undiagnosed dysuria/ pyuria – treat as if chlamydia
- Azithromycin 1 g orally
- If uncomplicated UTI – Bactrim® DS one orally twice daily × 7 days
- Pyridium® 200 mg po three times daily for 2 days
- If > 45 kg – can use 3 to 7 day course quinolones

Order renal ultrasound:

In adolescents with:

- Pyelonephritis
- Inadequate response to antibiotics
- Recurrent UTIs

Order voiding cystourethrogram (VCUG) or radionuclide cystogram:

In adolescents with:

- Abnormal renal ultrasound
- Family history of vesicoureteral reflux
- Clinical pyelonephritis

Order renal ultrasound/VCUG or radionuclide cystogram:

In children with:

- One or two UTIs
- IF patient admitted with pyelonephritis *or*
- IF 2 outpatient-treated uncomplicated UTIs

Order VCUG and renal ultrasound:

- IF diagnosed with urinary reflux, any grade

    Treat with antibiotic prophylaxis

    Bactrim® 2 mg/kg nightly

    Repeat VCUG/ renal ultrasound 1 year

    If no improvement – refer to urology

IF adolescent with recurrent UTI with negative VCUG and renal ultrasound:

Non-sexually active:

- Treat at first symptom with Macrobid® twice daily for 5 days

Sexually active

- Encourage voiding after intercourse
- Bactrim® 40/200 mg (half of a 80/400 mg tablet) within 2 hours of coitus

BIBLIOGRAPHY

Emans SJ. Vulvovaginal complaints in the adolescent. In Emans SJ, Laufer MR, Goldstein DP, eds. *Pediatric and Adolescent Gynecology,* 4th edn. Philadelphia: Lippincott-Raven, 1998:449–52

63 Uterine masses

NORMAL ULTRASOUND FINDINGS

Prepubertal: length 2 to 3.3 cm; width 0.5 to 1.0 cm; fundus = cervix size

Postpubertal: length 5 to 8 cm; width 1.6 to 3.0 cm; fundus > cervix size

ABNORMAL UTERINE FINDINGS

Fibroids (leiomyomas)

Rare in teenagers

If found, generally asymptomatic and should be left alone

Consider myomectomy in isolated, symptomatic, obstructive leiomyomas

Adenomyosis

Rare in teenagers

If symptomatic, difficult to treat as definitive treatment is hysterectomy

- Try suppression with continuous oral contraceptive (OCP)
- If OCP unsuccessful, try monthly GnRH agonist (Lupron Depot® 3.75 mg IM) for 6 months followed by continuous OCP

Polyps

Rare in teenagers

Symptom is persistent bleeding

If symptomatic, treat with hysteroscopic excision

Endometrial hyperplasia

Rare in teenagers

Associated with prolonged amenorrhea in the obese patient with polycystic ovarian syndrome

Diagnosed by endometrial biopsy or D&C when such a patient continues with breakthrough bleeding despite hormonal manipulation

Treatment as for adult with progestins

Mullerian anomalies:

Bicornuate uterus

- Associated other anomalies, skeletal and renal
- No issues in adolescence
- Counsel that may affect implantation of pregnancy and seek specialist if early loss or difficulty with conception

Unicornuate uterus

- Associated other anomalies, skeletal and renal
- May have increased dysmenorrhea; if occurs, use OCP

Uterine didelphys

- Associated other anomalies, skeletal and renal
- No issues in adolescence; counseling regarding potential of implantation in one or both horns
- Generally associated with two cervices; when becomes sexually active will need Pap test from each cervix

Obstructed hemi-uterus

- Associated other anomalies, skeletal and renal
- Usually obstructed on the right side and patent on the left
- Associated with intermittent pain that is not necessarily associated with the menstrual cycle
- Ultrasound and CT are not helpful in imaging; MRI best imaging modality
- Initial treatment is directed at conservation with continuous OCP; try ultra-low dose (20 µg), if unsuccessful, try higher estrogen doses

- Attempts at conservation are rare in the adolescent who is often not mature enough to tolerate the discomfort
- Definitive therapy is excision

    Usually well-defined fibrous septum between the two uteri and the uterus can be removed laparoscopically without entering the other one

    If there is no fibrous band, it may be best to excise by laparotomy to minimize any damage to the remaining uterus and reconstruct layers adequately; patient will need a Cesarean section in the future

Diethylstilbestrol (DES) abnormalities secondary to *in utero* exposure (last known exposure in US early 1980s)

T shaped appearance of the endometrial cavity; constricting bands in the cavity; hypoplasia; and synechiae

Cervix anomalies include:

- fibrous ridges
- hoods – circular fold that partially covers the cervix
- cock's comb – an irregular peak on the anterior border
- hypoplasia
- pseudopolyp

To date limited studies on second generation DES-exposed female offspring have shown no reproductive abnormalities/consequences

64 Uterovaginal agenesis/ androgen insensitivity

DIFFERENTIAL DIAGNOSIS

(See Figure 64-1)

Congenital absence of uterus and vagina

- Also called (Mayer-Rokitansky-Kuster-Hauser (MRKH) syndrome)
- Most common
- May have associated renal agenesis

Androgen insensitivity (AI)

Low-lying transverse vaginal septum

Agenesis of the lower 1/3rd of the vagina

Imperforate hymen

PRESENTATION

Typically as teenager with amenorrhea +/– cyclic abdominal pain

Incidental finding on well-child examination

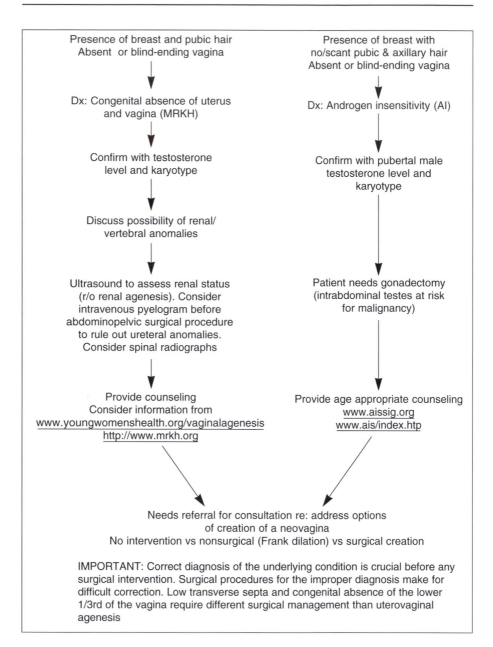

Figure 64-1 Algorithm for diagnosis of uterovaginal agenesis in the adolescent patient

DIAGNOSIS

History

Age – typical presentation age 15–18 years

Timing of pubertal development

- Breast/pubic hair

History of other congenital anomalies

- Cardiac, vertebral, tracheoesophageal

In the adolescent: cyclic abdominal pain – (consider presence of mullerian remnant/structure)

Physical examination

Pelvic assessment:

- Assess pubic hair development (AI patients may have sparse to no pubic hair)
- Check for vaginal opening
- Gently probe with lubricated cotton swab or male urethral swab/ 5 Fr pediatric feeding tube to assess introital patency/vaginal length
- Rectal exam

    Check for palpable cervix/uterine fundus/ovarian tissue

    Presence rules out AI/MRKH

Imaging

Consider pelvic ultrasound to confirm findings

- Presence of uterus rules out AI or MRKH

Consider MRI when ultrasound equivocal

- May be helpful to put cotton swab dipped in Crisco or a vitamin E capsule at perineum to define location of introitus

BIBLIOGRAPHY

Nonsurgical diagnosis and management of vaginal agenesis. Committee Opinion Number 274. American College of Obstetricians and Gynecologists. *Obstet Gynecol* 2002;100:213–16

65 Vaginal bleeding in the prepubertal patient

Most common causes:

> Foreign body
>
> Urethral prolapse
>
> Group B streptococcus vaginitis
>
> *Shigella* vaginitis
>
> Trauma

DIAGNOSIS

History

Age

Medical conditions:

> Recent sore throats/illnesses/medications including ingesting hormones

Recent/previous genital injury

Easy bruising, bleeding; family history of same

How long; more than once; just on toilet paper or on underwear; clots vs spotting

Physical examination

Height/weight measurements plotted on age appropriate curve (see Obesity, Chapter 35, for normal growth curves)

Vital signs; hemodynamic status

Thyroid enlargement

Axillary hair

Breast development

Abdominal enlargement

Bruising

Genitalia: estrogenized, discharge, blood, mass, foreign body, laceration

Laboratory tests

Evidence of thyroid disease: thyroid stimulating hormone, prolactin

Evidence of bruising: complete blood count with platelets, coagulation panel

Evidence of advanced puberty (see Puberty, Chapter 51)

Evidence of vaginal discharge, bleeding: vaginal aerobic, *Neisseria gonorrheae, Chlamydia trachomatis, Shigella* cultures

If all above negative: pelvic and renal ultrasound

MANAGEMENT

Evidence of vaginal discharge and/or bleeding: after obtaining the cultures as above, lavage the vagina with a 5 mm pediatric feeding tube attached to a 20 ml syringe filled with saline; avoid touching hymen during this process

Treat as tests above indicate

If all of the above negative and persists, schedule an exam under anesthesia (see Operative care, Chapter 37)

If exam under anesthesia normal consider pelvic MRI and if negative, referral or consultation with pediatric endocrinology

BIBLIOGRAPHY

Merritt DF. Evaluation of vaginal bleeding in the preadolescent. *Semin Pediatr Surg* 1998;7:35–42

66 Vaginal tract anomalies

Need to accurately define the anatomy of the pelvic organs prior to any planned surgical correction

It is very important to distinguish between a transverse vaginal septum versus cervical atresia, since incision into the uterus without adequate repair may lead to sepsis and possible mortality

SPECIFIC ANOMALIES

Imperforate hymen (see Hymenal anatomy, Chapter 25)

Transverse vaginal septum

Vaginal agenesis (see Uterovaginal agenesis/androgen insensitivity, Chapter 64)

Vaginal atresia

Cervical atresia

Longitudinal vaginal septum

Urogenital sinus

TRANSVERSE VAGINAL SEPTUM (TVS)

Definition

Failure in fusion and/or canalization of the urogenital sinus and mullerian ducts

Clinical presentation

Usually presents at the time of menarche with a history of cyclic abdominal pain and primary amenorrhea

May also present with urinary frequency or retention

May be diagnosed at time of well-child examination

May present with first speculum exam if previous spontaneous perforation already occurred

Physical examination

Findings may vary depending on the location of the transverse vaginal septum

The location of the septum may be:

- Low: Incidence 14%
                  As menstrual blood accumulates in the vagina there may be associated protrusion of the hymen. This protrusion usually does not move with Valsalva maneuver as it would with an imperforate hymen

- Midvagina: Incidence 40%
                  A blind vaginal pouch is encountered on pelvic examination. The transverse septum does not move with Valsalva maneuver

- Upper vagina: Incidence 46%
                  A deep blind vaginal pouch is encountered on pelvic examination. The thickness of the septum is usually thicker, approaching 1 cm in thickness when located closer to the cervix. The transverse septum does not move with the Valsalva maneuver

Pathophysiology

- May be associated with a female sex-limited autosomal recessive transmission
- Other reported Mendelian disorders:

  Amish population: transverse vaginal septum with congenital cataracts, severe scoliosis, unilateral absence of leg

  Transverse vaginal septum with congenital heart disease and post-axial polydactyly

Diagnosis

Ultrasound and/or MRI

- Need to determine thickness of septum
- Need to identify cervix to differentiate between high septum and congenital absence of cervix (cervical atresia – see below)

Intravenous pyelogram (IVP)

- Assciated renal anomalies are common

Treatment

General concepts

- Surgical excision of the transverse vaginal septum with the cut edges joined by an end-to-end anastomosis. The anastomosis may require undermining and mobilization of the vaginal mucosa
- If the TVS suspected prior to patient beginning her menses, it would be preferable to follow with close observation until menses to allow for definitive diagnosis of TVS differentiating from cervical or vaginal atresia and imperforate hymen
- To further decrease the thickness of the TVS, preoperative vaginal distention with dilators can thin the TVS and facilitate ease of septum excision

Specific treatment dependent on position of TVS

Utilize urinary catheter and finger in rectum to guide dissection of surgical plane

Use interrupted absorbable sutures for closure

Low:	Placement of a spinal needle through the septum with aspiration of the menstrual blood will verify the presence of TVS and direction of the axis of the vagina. Resection of septum followed by end-to-end anastomosis of upper and lower vaginal mucosa
Mid:	Distending vagina with vaginal dilators and waiting for menstrual blood to accumulate are important steps to miminize thickness of TVS. Z-plasty technique of septum removal may prevent post-repair vaginal stenosis
Upper:	Due to thickness of the TVS, should observe same techniques for midvaginal repair. May need to mobilize the vaginal tissue and rotate surgical flaps to cover vaginal defect. Vaginal mold with hollow core may need to be placed in vagina for wound healing

VAGINAL ATRESIA (VA)

Definition

Failure of the urogenital sinus to contribute to the lower portion of the vagina. The vagina is replaced by fibrous tissue above which well-developed mullerian structures are found (uterus, cervix and upper vagina)

Pathophysiology

Described genetic disorders

- VA with renal and middle ear anomalies
- VA with ossicle abnormalities of middle ear and renal dysgenesis

Clinical presentation

Primary amenorrhea with cyclic or chronic pain after menarche

Pelvic or abdominal mass with accumulation of blood in upper vagina

Physical findings

Normal secondary sexual characteristics

Vaginal dimple at introitus

Rectal exam reveals palpable upper vagina, cervix and uterus

Diagnosis

Ultrasound/MRI

IVP

Treatment

Best performed when a large hematocolpos present to assist in identification of defect

Consider preoperative dilator use as with TVS

Dissection is similar to that with transverse vaginal septum repair, once vaginal mucosa identified, a pull through procedure to bring vaginal tissue to hymenal opening is completed

CERVICAL ATRESIA

Diagnosis

Absence of upper vagina and cervix, very rare

Clinical presentation

The accumulation of menstrual blood in the uterine cavity leads to a history of cyclic abdominal pain and primary amenorrhea

Pelvic findings

On pelvic examination, can find a blind vaginal pouch with a small dimple at apex of the vagina

Diagnosis

Ultrasound – reveals distended uterus

MRI – can document presence or absence of cervical tissue and clarify pelvic anatomy

Treatment

Medical

Can suppress menses with continuous oral contraceptives either long-term or while awaiting definitive surgical procedure

Surgical excision

Surgical creation of cervical os has been reported but is difficult due to large amount of absent tissue and difficulty in maintaining post-operative patent opening to uterus; therefore, hysterectomy often necessary to prevent intervening infection with possible fatal sepsis

Due to uncommon nature of anomaly, referral to regional expert with prior experience is strongly recommended

LONGITUDINAL VAGINAL SEPTUM (LVS)

Definition

Intravaginal tissue arising from abnormal mesodermal proliferation or persistence of epithelium during canalization separating the vagina into two distinct cavities; may occur in either a coronal or sagittal orientation

Pathophysiology

Rarely can be a genetic association

LVS with aplastic nasal ala, microcephaly, deafness, hypothyroidism, skeletal dysplasia and gastrointestinal malabsorption

Clinical presentation

Presentations vary based on extent of LVS present

- Two vaginal canals with two separate cervical openings

  Patient may be asymptomatic. Often the vaginal septum is pushed to one side and only one vaginal canal with one cervix present upon cursory pelvic exam

- One vaginal canal present with occlusion of the second canal by fusion of the vaginal septum to the vagina, creating a hemivagina

  Presentation is often variable depending upon the extent of the hemivagina. If the vaginal septum is perforated, amount of accumulated blood will be less. If more menstrual cycles occur, additional blood accumulates in the hemivagina often leading to the formation of a pelvic mass. This is part of a well-recognized malformation called uterine didelphys with obstructed hemivagina and ipsilateral renal agenesis and occurs more frequently on the right

Diagnosis

Ultrasound/MRI

Treatment

Surgical excision of the longitudinal vaginal septum

- If a longitudinal septum is present without vaginal occlusion, the septum does not need excision
- Indications for excision:

  Interference with intercourse

  Difficulty with tampon use

  Inability to visualize both cervices for Pap testing

- If obstructed hemivagina:

    Place large bore angiocath through vaginal bulge to identify blocked upper vagina, then dilate created opening with clamp. Grasp edges of septum and excise excess septal tissue, reapproximating edges with absorbable suture ensuring opening wide enough to permit visualization of cervix

UROGENITAL SINUS

Definition

Persistence of the common urogenital canal with a normal anus and rectum

Etiology

Congenital adrenal hyperplasia (CAH)

Diagnosis

Visual inspection of perineum:

Anal opening is in normal position with a single perineal orifice anteriorly

May be associated with clitoromegaly if due to CAH

Imaging

Confirmed with genitogram (see Radiologic imaging for gynecologic conditions, Chapter 52)

MRI – to rule out associated lumbosacral anomalies, tethered cord

Renal ultrasound – to rule out associated renal anomalies

Cystoscopy under anesthesia

Treatment

Surgical correction varies upon level at which urethra and vagina converge

Correction should be done in consultation with pediatric surgery

Medical management includes treatment of underlying endocrinopathy, if present (e.g. CAH)

BIBLIOGRAPHY

Edwards DK, Muram D. Sexual developmental anomalies and their reconstruction: Upper and lower tracts. In Sanfilippo JS, Muram D, Dewhurst J, Lee PA, eds. *Pediatric and Adolescent Gynecology*, 2nd edn. Philadelphia: WB Saunders & Co, 2001

Garcia RF. Z-plasty correction for congenital transverse vaginal septum. *Am J Obstet Gynecol* 1967;99:1164

Hendren WH. Urogenital sinus and cloacal malformation. *Semin Pediatr Surg* 1996;5:72–9

Laufer MR, Goldstein DP. Structural anomalies of the female reproductive tract. In Emans JS, Laufer MR, Goldstein DP, eds. *Pediatric and Adolescent Gynecology*, 4th edn. Philadelphia: Lippincott-Raven, 1998

Rock JA, Jones HW. The double uterus associated with an obstructed hemivagina and ipsilateral renal agenesis. *Am J Obstet Gynecol* 1980;138:339–42

Suidan FG, Azoury RS. The transverse vaginal septum: A clinicopathologic evaluation. *Obstet Gynecol* 1979;54:278–83

67 Vulvar nevi

Uncommon to find vulvar nevi in children/adolescents

Most darkly pigmented vulvar lesions in this age group are lentigines (benign freckle-like increases in the concentration of melanocytes in the basal layer of the epithelium) or are benign nevi

TYPES

Benign nevi

    Junctional nevi: small 2–10 mm diameter

- Flat with minimal elevation above skin surface
- Involve only epidermis/dermis junction
- Uniform color from tan–black
- Well-demarcated, smooth contour
- Can be monitored every 6–12 months
- Biopsy with color/surface or size change

    Compound nevi: arise from compound nevi or *de novo*

- Involve epidermis and dermis
- Size 4–10 mm diameter
- Uniform color/regular margins
- May become papular/polypoid/pedunculated

        And when change occurs consider excisional biopsy

Melanoma

    Rare in children/teens especially on the vulva

    80% cases in children have no predisposing factors

    Second most common neoplasm of the vulva

RISK FACTORS

For childhood melanoma:

Congenital melanocytic nevi

Dysplastic nevi

Xeroderma pigmentosum

Immunosuppression

DIAGNOSIS

History

Duration of lesion

Change in lesion

Size, color, bleeding

Family history of melanoma

Physical examination

Perform thorough skin assessment for lesions

Avoid just identifying lesion of concern

Identify lesion of concern

MANAGEMENT

Perform excisional biopsy for any irregular, bleeding, palpable, large lesions or for those of concern to family (> 3 mm) (see Operative care, Chapter 37)

When uncertain refer to pediatric dermatology for opinion

Follow-up and manage based on microscopic pathology results

BIBLIOGRAPHY

Egan CA, Bradley RR, Logsdon VK, *et al*. Vulvar melanoma in childhood. *Arch Dermatol* 1997;133:345–8

Rock B, Hood AF, Rock JA. Prospective study of vulvar nevi. *J Am Acad Dermatol* 1990;22:104–6

Schroeder B. Vulvar disorders in adolescents. *Obstet Gynecol Clin North Am* 2000;27:35–48

68 Vulvar ulcers

Infectious

Coxsackie A16:

> Group of blisters or red spots can occur on the buttocks, genitalia and/or extremities

Epstein–Barr virus (EBV):

> Rare association of single or multiple painful ulcers with infectious mononucleosis

Streptococcus:

> Single painful shallow ulcer

Varicella:

> Same as herpes simplex but rare except in immunocompromised state

Sexually transmitted diseases (STDs)

Chancroid:

> One or more painful ulcers with regional lymphadenopathy

Granuloma inguinale (donovanosis):

> Painless, progressive ulcerative without regional lymphadenopathy. Lesions are highly vascular (beefy red) and bleed easily on contact

Herpes simplex:

> see Sexually transmitted diseases, Chapter 56

Lymphogranuloma venereum (LGV):

> Tender inguinal and/or femoral adenopathy that is usually unilateral, sometimes associated with a self-limited ulcer

Syphilis:

See Sexually transmitted diseases, Chapter 56

Systemic diseases

Apthous ulcers:

Single or multiple deep painful ulcers of the labia minora and occasionally the oral pharynx; associated with a upper respiratory infection or other viral syndromes

Behcet's syndrome:

Multisystem involvement that includes arthritis, uveitis and mucocutaneous lesions of the eyes, mouth and genitalia. Painful, shallow, crisp borders (like a hole punch), persistent ulcers commonly on the labia minora and occasionally on the oropharynx

Crohn's disease:

Single or multiple deep painful ulcers of the perineum which may or may not have associated anal and perianal lesions of skin tags, fissures, fistulas, ulcers and abscesses

Autoimmune diseases

Bullous pemphigoid:

Single or grouped vesicular lesions that are painful which may or may not be associated with similar lesions on face, neck, palms and soles

Chronic bullous disease of childhood:

Annular arrangement of tense vesicles/bullae with strong predilection for perineum which may be associated with similar oral lesions (60%) and ocular symptoms (40%). Usually remits before puberty

Kawasaki disease:

Bright erythema, with edema sometimes followed by desquamation

Systemic lupus erythematosus (SLE):

Erythema progresses to macular eruptions and/or fissures leading to ulcerations

Cutaneous drug reactions

Erythema multiforme

Painful oral and genital ulcers accompanied by target-like lesions on the palms, soles and other parts of the body

No prodrome

Lesions last on average a week

Precipitated by an allergic reaction to a medication or preceded by herpes simplex

Stevens–Johnson syndrome

Similar skin reactions as erythema multiforme but more severe mucous membrane involvement with possible necrosis

Prodrome 1–14 days: fever, headache, sore throat, malaise, coughing, vomiting and/or diarrhea

Lesions last on average a week

Precipitated by medications (NSAIDs, sulfonamides, and anticonvulsants), herpes simplex, and mycoplasma pneumonia

Toxic epidermal necrolysis (TEN)

Sudden destruction of skin and mucosa; 20–30% risk of death

Precipitated by a variety of medications including the ones that cause Stevens–Johnson syndrome

Long-term sequelae:

- Vulvar synechiae and/or atrophy
- Vestibular or introital stenosis
- Adhesions upper 2/3rd vagina

DIAGNOSIS

Child

Thorough medical, surgical, and social history; complete physical exam including all mucous membranes, hands and feet, and external inspection of anus and genitalia

Culture for streptococcus, other aerobes, herpes, and *Chlamydia*

If negative, check complete blood count (CBC) with differential and erythrocyte sedimentation rate (ESR) to rule out viral, immunologic, gastrointestinal or dermatologic condition; check rapid plasma reagin to rule out syphilis

If still negative and persists with local measures, consider biopsy

Most biopsies of the genitalia in children need to be done with anesthesia (see Operative care, Chapter 37)

Adolescent

Thorough medical, surgical, gynecologic and social history; complete physical exam including all mucous membranes, hands and feet, and external inspection of anus and genitalia

Culture for streptococcus, other aerobes, herpes, and *Chlamydia*

If negative, check CBC, ESR to rule out viral, immunologic, gostrointestinal or dermatologic conditions; check monospot (may have a 7–14 day lag from symptoms to diagnosis) or EBV titres to rule out Epstein–Barr virus; check eye exam to rule out uveitis seen in Bechet's syndrome

If negative, consider treatment with sitz baths and if symptomatic topical clobetasol ointment bid

If does not regress or recurs, consider biopsy:

> Place EMLA cream (see EMLA^R use, Chapter 17)
>
> Use a vulvar punch to the depth of the dermis and to a width that includes normal and abnormal cells
>
> Attain hemostasis with silver nitrate or a 4-0 chromic suture
>
> Encourage healing with tid sitz baths
>
> Ice and oral Advil for analgesia

MANAGEMENT

(See Table 68-1 for list of appropriate corticosteroid ointments)

Infectious

Coxsackie A16

Medications:

> Try emollients such as A&D, Desitin; if fails try topical OTC steroid ointment in conjunction with topical xylocaine bid; overall not typically helpful

Course:

> May need to urinate in a sitz bath but rarely causes urinary retention
>
> Sitz baths/ice for comfort
>
> Viral course that can involve hand, foot and mouth as well (called hand, foot and mouth disease); fever lasts up to 4 days; genital ulcers about 7 days

Table 68-1 Steroid ointment dosing (ointment preferred as non-alcohol base)
See Stoughton (1989) for more complete list

	Brand name	*Generic name*
Ultra-high	Temovate® (0.05%)	Clobetasol (0.05%)
Mid-potency	Cutivate®	Fluticasone (0.005%)
	Synalar®(0.025%)	Triamcinolone (0.025%)
		Hydrocortisone (2.0%)
Low potency	Aclovate®(0.05%)	Aclometasone (0.05%)
		Hydrocortisone (1.0%) OTC

Epstein–Barr Virus (EBV)

Medications

Topical ultra-potent steroid ointment (i.e. clobetasol) in conjunction with topical xylocaine bid

Course

May need to urinate in a sitz bath but rarely causes urinary retention

Sometimes is associated with a fever and/or non-specific viral infection

Local care as with herpes

Streptococcus

Local care: sitz baths 3–4 × a day; minimize irritants and rubbing

Antibiotic for ten days:

Amoxicillin 20–50 mg/kg/24 h/3 doses po

Ampicillin 50–100 mg/kg/24 h/4 doses po (not to exceed 2–4 g/24 h)

Cephalexin 25–50 mg/kg/24 h/2–4 doses po

Erythromycin 30–50 mg/kg/24 h/3–4 doses po (not to exceed 2 g/24 h)

Over 45 kg use adult dose

Varicella

Same medical and local treatment as for herpes simplex

Atarax® for itching 2 mg/kg/24 h div q 6 h

Watch for secondary infection, i.e. impetigo from scratching

STDs

Chancroid

Medication

Azithromycin 1 g orally in a single dose *or*

Ceftriaxone 250 mg IM

Ciprofloxacin 500 mg orally bid for 3 days

Erythromycin base 500 mg po tid for 7 days

Course

If treatment is successful ulcers usually improve symptomatically within 3 days and objectively within 7 days after therapy

Time for healing depends on the size of the ulcer; large ulcers may take 2 weeks or longer

Clinical resolution of fluctuant lymphadenopathy is slower than that of ulcers and if still symptomatic may require needle aspiration or incision and drainage

Granuloma inguinale (Donovanosis)

Medications

Doxycycline 100 mg po bid for at least three weeks

Trimethoprim sulfate DS one po bid for at least three weeks

or until lesions heal

Course

Lesions may have secondary bacterial infection or may be co-infected with another STD

Treatment halts progression of lesions but prolonged therapy may be required until ulcers completely resolve

Herpes simplex

(see Sexually transmitted diseases, Chapter 56)

LGV

Medication: Doxycycline 100 mg po bid × 21 days; alternative erythromycin base 500 mg po qid × 21 days

Buboes may require I&D to prevent formation of inguinal/femoral lacerations; consult pediatric infectious disease

Syphilis

(see Sexually transmitted diseases, Chapter 56)

Systemic diseases

Aphthous ulcers

Medications

> Topical ultra-potent steroid ointment (i.e. clobetasol) in conjunction with topical lidocaine jelly bid

Course

> Local care as with herpes

> May need to urinate in a sitz bath but rarely causes urinary retention

> Sometimes is associated with a fever and/or non-specific viral infection

> May recur

Behcet's syndrome

Medications

> Topical ultra-potent steroid ointment (i.e. clobetasol) in conjunction with topical xylocaine bid

Course

> Local care as with herpes

> May need to urinate in a sitz bath but rarely causes urinary retention

> If course is prolonged consult pediatric dermatology and/or rheumatology

> May be the only sign of the syndrome initially but recurrences will eventually be associated with other signs

Crohn's disease

Medications

> Topical ultra-potent steroid ointment (i.e. clobetasol) in conjunction with topical xylocaine bid

Course

> Local care as with herpes

> Resolution with treatment of the bowel disease

> Treatment should be undertaken in consultation with pediatric gastroenterology

Kawasaki and SLE

Local care: frequent soaks, analgesia – topical and systemic

Treat the particular systemic disease more aggressively

If unsuccessful consult with pediatric dermatology

Autoimmune diseases

Bullous pemphigoid

Medications

Topical corticosteroid ointment, medium potency (i.e. hydrocortisone 2.0%)

Course

Should be managed in consultation with pediatric dermatology

Chronic bullous disease of childhood

Medications

Dapsone® +/– systemic steroids

Course

Should be managed in consultation with pediatric dermatology

Cutaneous drug reactions

For Stevens–Johnson and TEN: aggressive fluid and electrolyte management, local care as for burn patient; expect reepithelialization in 2–3 weeks, mucous membrane resolution may take months

BIBLIOGRAPHY

Fivozinsky KB, Laufer MR. Vulvar disorders in adolescents. *Adolesc Med* 1999;10:305–19

Ridley CM. Vulvar disease in the pediatric population. *Semin Dermatol* 1996;15:29–35

CDC Sexually Transmitted Diseases Treatment Guidelines 2002. *MMWR* 2002;51(RR-6)

Stoughton RB. Percutaneous absorption of drugs. *Annu Rev Pharmacol Toxicol* 1989;29:55–69 (Complete table of topical corticosteroids)

Wilkinson EJ, Stone IK. *Atlas of Vulvar Disease*. Baltimore: Williams and Wilkins; 1995

69 Vulvovaginitis

PEDIATRIC PATIENT

KEY POINTS

Most common gynecologic complaint in prepubertal girl

Typical complaint is discharge, dysuria, pruritis, or vulvar redness

Most cases are 'non-specific vulvovaginitis' without a specific infectious etiology

Cases with an infectious cause tend to have visible discharge and vulvar erythema

Most cases respond to hygienic and supportive measures

Candida or yeast is an uncommon pathogen in the toilet-trained prepubertal girl

Definition

Inflammation of vulva and vaginal tissues

In children, vulva may be inflamed first with vagina uninvolved or vulva may be secondarily affected

Risk factors

Anatomic

- Lack of labial fat pads and pubic hair
- Thin, sensitive vulvar skin
- Thin, atrophic vaginal epithelium
- Prepubertal hypoestrogenic vagina has a neutral pH and is an excellent bacterial culture medium

Hygiene

- Poor hand washing
- Inadequate cleansing of vulva after voiding or bowel movements
- Exposure to vulvar irritants (e.g. dirt, sand, soaps)

Foreign body

Sexual abuse

DIAGNOSIS

History

Purpose: To distinguish between vulvitis (e.g. erythematous, itching vulva) and vaginitis (e.g. discharge)

- Try to direct questioning to child/patient as much as possible

When did complaints begin?

- Symptoms present for months/years – likely to be non-specific etiology
- Short duration of symptoms < 1 month – more likely to be specific bacterial etiology

Color of the discharge: white, yellow, green, purulent, or bloody

- *Bloody* discharge – think foreign body, *Shigella*, group A beta-hemolytic streptococci, trauma, vulvar scratching, condyloma, rarely precocious puberty or tumor
- *Green* discharge think of specific causes like *Staphylococcus* or *Streptococcus*, *Haemophilus influenzae*, gonorrhea, or foreign body

Does the discharge have any odor?

- Foul-smelling discharge – associated with foreign body (e.g. toilet paper), vaginitis

Ask about:

- What treatments or medicines have been used to treat condition
- Use of bubble baths
- What type of soaps and shampoos used – Ivory and Dial very harsh
- Any symptoms of anal pruritus – associated with pinworm infestation

- History of any skin conditions: atopic dermatitis, eczema
- History of recent upper respiratory/pharyngeal/skin infections in patient or family

Any clues/concerns about sexual abuse: behavioral changes, nightmares

Have child answer questions:

- Do you have itching, pain before or after itching?
- Do you have to change your panties or underwear frequently because of the discharge?

    If so, how often?

Perineal hygiene: Have patient demonstrate wiping after bowel movement: front-to-back or back-to-front

Physical examination

Perform general physical exam

- Look for evidence skin conditions: psoriasis, eczema
- Look for evidence bruising, trauma – evidence of abuse
- Assess for secondary sexual characteristics: breast budding/axillary hair

Inspect external genitalia: perineum, vulva and vagina

- Look for erythema, discharge, excoriations, ulcers, condyloma, tumors
- Use labial traction to allow better visualization of vagina (see Gynecologic examination, Chapter 21)
- Consider use of knee–chest position to allow complete assessment of vagina (see Gynecologic examination, Chapter 21)

    May be able to visualize upper vagina and may be helpful to rule out foreign body

IF discharge present:

Use Dacron male urethral swabs to obtain specimens

- Aerobic culture
- Cultures for gonorrhea and *Chlamydia*
- Wet mount when able to obtain third sample

    Yeast and *Trichomonas* are not commonly found in the prepubertal patient, yeast not common outside the diaper period unless recent use of antibiotics.

Trichomonas is rare and sexually transmitted (see Sexual abuse, Chapter 54)

Bacterial vaginosis is rare in the prepubertal child. While not sexually transmitted, it is more common in sexual abuse, follow carefully and look for other indicators

- IF no discharge AND no response to previous routine hygiene measures:

  Use small pediatric feeding tube attached to syringe or catheter within a catheter technique (as described in Gynecologic examination, Chapter 21) to put one or two drops of fluid into vagina and aspirate for specimens

- After obtaining specimens for culture, IF suspect foreign body:

  Use small pediatric feeding tube attached to 20 ml syringe filled with warm water. Use labial traction to allow hymen to open, and gently place feeding tube through vagina without touching hymen and try to flush out foreign body from vagina

Rectoabdominal exam (optional)

- May allow practitioner to express a discharge from the vagina not previously seen, allow palpation of hard foreign bodies or detect abnormal masses

Diagnosis

Non-specific vulvovaginitis

- Erythematous vulva:
- Culture grows normal flora or Gram-negative enteric bacteria (e.g. *Escherichia coli, Enterococcus*)

Specific causes

- Determined by culture results

MANAGEMENT

Non-specific vulvitis/vulvovaginitis:

Educate caregiver: use Pediatric vulvovaginitis pamphlet (North American Society for Pediatric and Adolescent Gynecology. Tel: 215-955-6331)

Improved hygiene:

- White cotton underpants/cotton crotch
- Front-to-back wiping

- Good hand washing

- Urinate with legs apart to limit urine reflux into vagina

- Avoid vulvar skin irritants (bubble baths)

- Shampoo hair while standing in shower to avoid sitting in dirty, soapy water

- Wear loose-fitting skirts; avoid tight clothing

Sitz bath in warm tap water – 15 min 2 to 3 times daily

Bland soap when bathing (such as unscented Dove or Basis)

Avoid soap to vulva

Pat vulva dry or dry with blow dryer on cool setting

Apply protective barrier cream to vulva (e.g. Destin, A & D ointment or Aqua-phor®)

If no response in 48 h:

- Reexamine patient

- Exclude pinworms or empiric treatment with mebendazole

- Empiric treatment with amoxicillin, amoxicillin clavualnate or cephalosporin for 10 days

    or

- Rarely need vulvar biopsy under anesthesia if vulva still erythematous

Persistent non-specific vulvovaginitis:

Options:

10–14 day course oral antibiotics such as amoxicillin, amoxicillin clavulanate or cephalosporin

1 month course of nightly dose of amoxicillin clavulanate, cephalexin, or trimethoprim/sulfamethoxazole

1 week use of topical antibacterial cream use (e.g. mupirocin)

Course of nightly applied small amount estrogen-containing cream (e.g. Premarin or Estrace:

   Watch for signs of systemic absorption (e.g. breast budding), if occurs discontinue the cream

Emphasize continued hygiene measures

Consider examination under anesthesia

Table 69-1 Specific causes and treatment of vulvovaginitis

Etiology	Drug	Dose	Route	Duration
Streptococcus pyogenes	Penicillin V	250 mg TID	po	10 days
Haemophilus influenzae	Amoxicillin	20–40 mg/kg/day divided q 8 hrs	po	10 days
For resistant strains	Amoxicillin/ clavulanate	20–40 mg/kg/day divided q 8 hrs	po	7–10 days
	Trimethoprim– sulfamethoxazole	8 mg/40 mg/kg/day divided q 12 h	po	10 days
Staphylococcus aureus	Cephalexin	25–50 mg/kg/day divided q 12 hrs	po	7–10 days
	Dicloxacillin	25 mg/kg/day	po	7–10 days
	Amoxicillin/ clavulanate	20–40 mg/kg/day divided q 8 h	po	7–10 days
	Cefuroxime axetil susp	30 mg/kg/day bid (max 1 g)	po	10 days
	Cefuroxime axetil tabs	250 mg bid	po	10 days
Streptococcus pneumoniae	Penicillin	500 mg qid	po	10 days
	Erythromycin	50 mg/kg/day divided q 6 h	po	10days
	Trimethoprim– sulfamethoxazole	8 mg/40 mg/kg/day divided q 12 h	po	10 days
	Clarithromycin	15 mg/kg/day divided q 12 h	po	10 days
Shigella	Trimethoprim– sulfamethoxazole	8 mg/40 mg/kg/day divided q 12 h	po	10 days
For resistant strains	Cefixime	8 mg/kg/day single dose per day	po	10 days
	Cetriaxone	50 mg/kg/single IM dose (max 1 g)		
If > 45 kg:	Ciprofloxacin	250–500 mg q 12 h	po	7–14 days
	Azithromycin	1000 mg po 1st day, then 500 mg po q day × 4 days	po	
Chlamydia trachomatis	Erythromycin	50 mg/kg/day	po	10–14 days
	Azithromycin	20 mg/kg (max 1 g)	po	one dose
If > age 8 years	Doxycycline	100 mg bid	po	7 days
Neisseria gonorrheae	Ceftriaxone	125 mg	IM	one dose
Candida	Nystatin		topical	7 days
	Miconazole		topical	7 days
	Clotrimazole		topical	7 days
	Terconazole		topical	7 days
Trichomonas	Metronidazole	15 mg/kg/day tid (max 250 mg tid)	po	7–10 days
Pinworms	Mebendazole	1–100 mg tablet chewable po repeat in 2 wks		

Modified with permission from Emans SJ, Laufer MR, Goldstein DP, eds.
Pediatric Adolescent Gynecology, 4th edn. Philadelphia: Lippincott-Raven Publishers, 1998;88

ADOLESCENT PATIENT

KEY POINTS

Physiologic leukorrhea (normal estrogen related desquamation of epithelial cells) is the most common discharge in pubescent girl

Specific causes are more common in the adolescent

Vaginal discharge may be the presenting symptom for sexually transmitted diseases in the adolescent

With foul-smelling or bloody discharge think foreign body (most commonly a retained tampon)

DIAGNOSIS

Symptoms

Vaginal discharge, vulvar and/or vaginal itching/burning

Physical examination

Perform routine overall skin assessment:

- Look for signs of eczema, psoriasis, skin conditions

Inspect external genitalia:

- Look for erythema, discharge, excoriations, vesicles, and ulcers
- Evaluate vaginal discharge

   In virginal adolescents:

   May omit speculum exam

   Use saline-moistened cotton-tipped applicator or Dacron urethral swabs inserted just inside the hymenal ring to obtain specimens

   Perform pH testing:

   pH > 4.5: bacterial vaginosis or trichomoniasis

   pH < 4.5: physiologic leukorrhea or candida

   Perform wet mount

   Small amount of discharge on two slides

Normal saline slide:

Look for trichomonads

Look for clue cells (squamous epithelial cells whose borders are coated with adherent bacteria)

10% KOH slide (lyses squamous cell walls)

Look for hyphal elements of yeast

Perform whiff test:

Smell KOH slide to detect 'fishy' or amine odor indicating bacterial vaginosis

If patient is/has been sexually active or foul smelling or bloody discharge

- Look at vagina and cervix with speculum

Is there a foreign body or retained tampon?

Does cervical discharge appear purulent?

Is the cervix friable in appearance?

Perform endocervical testing for *Chlamydia*/gonorrhea

MANAGEMENT

(See Figure 69-1)

Physiologic leukorrhea

Etiology:

Normal vaginal epithelial desquamation secondary to estrogenization

Symptoms:

Clear, white discharge, wetness

Diagnosis:

Normal vaginal pH < 4.5 and wet mount without inflammation

Treatment:

Education: most teens are unaware of the cyclic nature and impact of hormonal changes on vaginal discharge; typically self-limited condition

Supportive: Encourage use of panty liners or shields

- Discourage use of douching attempts to clear normal process
- Occasionally oral contraceptives may help if menstruating

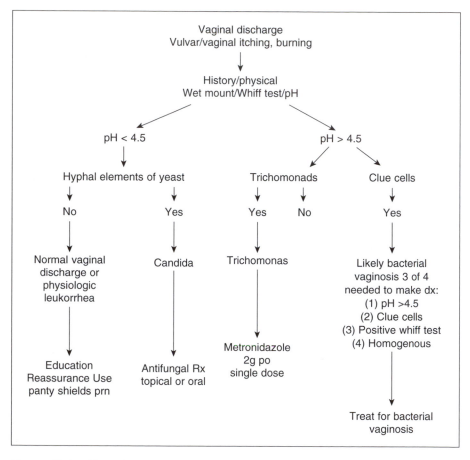

Figure 69-1 Algorithm for management of vaginal discharge in the adolescent

Candidal vaginitis

Etiology:

Yeast species are a part of normal vaginal flora

Infections result from overgrowth

Candida albicans, Torulopsis glabrata, Candida tropicalis

Risk factors:

Recent use antibiotics, diabetes

Symptoms:

Thick, white-yellow, clumped, pruritic discharge

Diagnosis:

History: Vulvovaginal pruritis, burning, may be worse post-coital, with urination

Exam: White, 'cheesy' discharge

- Erythematous vulva
- May have satellite red pustules or even raw, denuded areas from scratching
- May have fissuring at perineum, junction of labia

Tests: pH < 4.5 normal

- 10% KOH slide of wet mount shows mycelial forms/hyphae/budding yeast
- Can do culture on Biggy agar or Sabouraud agar

Treatment:

Initial:

- Topical antifungals: see Table 69-2
- Oral antifungal – fluconazole: see Table 69-2

Recurrent:

Fluconazole 100 mg po once/week for 6 months monitor liver function tests

Boric acid capsules 600 mg per vagina once/day for 14 days

Bacterial vaginosis

Etiology:

Increased concentration of normally occurring anaerobic vaginal organisms (*Gandnerella vaginalis*, *Bacteroides* and *Mobiluncus* species)

Diagnosis:

History: Malodorous discharge (may be worse after menses, coitus)

Exam: Thin, grey, malodorous discharge

Tests: Need 3 of 4 criteria

(1) pH > 4.5

2) Positive Whiff test

(3) Clue cells on wet mount

(4) Homogeneous discharge

Table 69-2   Treatment for candidiasis

Type	Brand Name	Dosing
Intravaginal methods		
Butaconazole 2% cream	Femstat*	1 applicatorful (5 g) for 3 nights
Clotrimazole 1% cream	Gyne-Lotrimin*	1 applicatorful (5 g) for 7 nights
	Mycelex-7*	1 applicatorful (5 g) for 7 nights
Clotrimazole vaginal tablets	Gyne-Lotrimin vaginal inserts*	100-mg vaginal tablet for 7 nights
		200-mg vaginal tablets for 3 nights
	Mycelex-G vaginal tablets	500-mg vaginal tablet for 1 night
Miconazole 2% cream	Monistat-7*	1 applicatorful (5 g) for 7 nights
Miconazole suppositories	Monistat-7*	100-mg vaginal suppository for 7 nights
	Monistat-3*	200-mg vaginal suppository for 3 nights
Terconazole 0.4% cream	Terazol 7	1 applicatorful (5 g) for 7 nights
Terconazole 0.8% cream	Terazol 3	1 applicatorful (5 g) or 3 nights
Terconazole suppositories	Terazol 3	30-mg vaginal suppository for 3 nights
Tioconazole 6.5% ointment	Vagistat-1	1 applicatorful (4.6 g) for 1 night
Oral methods		
Fluconazole oral tablets	Diflucan	One 150-mg tablet

*Available over the counter

Treatment:

Oral: Metronidazole 500 mg twice a day for 7 days

Clindamycin 300 mg twice a day for 7 days

Topical: Metronidazole gel 0.75%, one applicatorful (5 g) intravaginally once or twice a day for 7 days

Clindamycin cream 2%, one applicatorful (5 g) intravaginally at bedtime for 7 days

Trichomonas vaginalis

Etiology:

Trichomonas vaginalis, a small motile flagellated parasite

Sexually transmitted

Diagnosis:

History:	Discharge (frothy, malodorous, white or yellow)
	May have itching, dysuria, post-coital bleeding
	May be asymptomatic and found on Pap smear or wet prep
Exam:	Frothy, yellow-green or gray-white discharge
	Grossly visible punctate hemorrhages of the cervix (strawberry cervix) 2–10%
Test:	Wet prep reveals mobile flagellated organisms and increased amount of white blood cells
Treatment:	Metronidazole 2 g orally in one dose
	Sexual partner must also be treated with same medicine at same time
	Warn patient about anatabuse-like side-effects with metronidazole

        Nausea, vomiting, metallic aftertaste

        Avoid alcohol for 24–48 h after taking metronidazole to avoid associated nausea, vomiting

As *Trichomonas* is sexually transmitted, screen also for gonorrhea and *Chlamydia*

For resistant strains, consider ordering metronidazole susceptibility testing through the CDC: www.CDC.gov

BIBLIOGRAPHY

Baiulescu M, Hannon PR, Marcinak JF, *et al*. Chronic vulvovaginitis caused by antibiotic-resistant *Shigella flexneri* in a prepubertal child. *Pediatr Infect Dis* 2002;21:170–2

CDC. Sexually transmitted diseases treatment guidelines 2002. *MMWR* 2002;51 (RR-6)

Emans SJ. Vulvovaginal problems in the prepubertal child. In Emans JS, Laufer MR, Goldstein DP, eds. *Pediatric and Adolescent Gynecology*, 4th edn. Philadelphia: Lippincott-Raven, 1998:75–108

Jaquiery A, Stylianopoulos A, Hogg G, *et al*. Vulvovaginitis: clinical feature, aetiology and microbiology of the genital tract. *Arch Dis Child* 1999;81:64–7